MY BODY, MY VEHICLE

Your Atlas for Cruising the Highway to Health

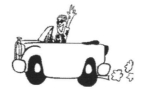

KELLIE CREAMER

This book was created with thoughtful preparation. It is intended as a guide to help you make the best choices for obtaining and maintaining a healthy, well balanced lifestyle. It is not designed in any way to be a prescription or substitution for treatment or medical care. You are strongly advised to get medical attention if you think you have a serious condition. None of this information is a replacement for any information your physician or dietician may have prescribed.

This book includes bibliographical references and an index. The books referenced are recommended as further reading if you desire more information to help steer you on the highway to health.

Cover illustration: Valters Verners
Editing: Helen Arnestad

Table of Contents

Introduction

The greatest wealth is health ~ Virgil

My Body, My Vehicle is a lifestyle and wellness book that focuses on the human body and how to treat it well, so that, in turn, your body treats you well. I wrote this book to share information about your body, how to respect it, feed it, move it, love it, and let it serve you to its fullest potential.

In this time of climate change and economic uncertainty, it is more important than ever for us humans to live in harmony with ourselves, with each other, and with our bodies. I believe that by slowly incorporating healthy food and lifestyle choices you can make a difference in yourself, and, ultimately, the world.

America's health is declining and our children are taking the brunt of it. Within the 20 years from the 1970's to 1990's, the percent of overweight children aged six to 11 doubled (from seven to 15 percent) and tripled for adolescents aged 12 to 19 (from five to 15 percent). Those numbers climb higher and higher each year as more children become obese. Recent reports indicate that children born today are the first generation in the history of America to have a shorter life expectancy than their parents! This is due to the obesity epidemic.

Today's adult Americans already have a shorter life expectancy than originally projected because of obesity. Currently, a staggering 64.5% of adults aged 20 and older are overweight and 30.5% are obese, that means one third of our adult population is obese! The percent of morbidly obese adults has tripled since 1990 to 6%. In a recent address, the Surgeon General announced that smoking is no longer the number one killer in the U.S. Obesity has replaced it!

Obesity in itself is not officially considered a disease, but it can trigger a number of other diseases, which this book will detail. One of the diseases is Type 2 Diabetes. The saddest and most harsh aspect of the obesity epidemic in children is that they are now subject to Type 2 Diabetes. When I was studying nutrition fifteen years ago, Type 2 Diabetes was referred to as Adult Onset Diabetes, which was its common name for generations, because it only happened in overweight adults with a sedentary lifestyle. Within the past ten years, Adult Onset was switched to its clinical name, Type 2, because so many children are getting this disorder. It is a serious, deadly, and debilitating disease that must be reduced in our nation.

We can help reverse these harsh statistics! The good news is that the triggered diseases are curable. Dr. Dean Ornish published studies indicating simple diet and lifestyle changes can reverse severe diseases such as heart disease (angina), Type 2 diabetes, prostate and breast cancer. It's a matter of choice and lifestyle. Too many of today's American food options are polluted with preservatives, flavor enhancers, trans-fats, additives, sugars and uber-sugars (like high fructose corn syrup). In addition, how can a population not be overweight when much of the meat and milk it consumes contains added growth hormones and growth enhancers? It's not impossible to imagine that some of those items are seeping into our bodies and enhancing our growth, is it?

Think of your body as your vehicle. If you lived thousands, or even one hundred years ago, your body would have been your vehicle. You would have been forced to move it without external help to fuel (or feed) it. You would have relied more on your intuitions and motivations and been more reliant on what was available from nature. Now, we have big grocery stores, fast food joints and convenience markets from which to obtain our nourishment. Your surroundings may have changed, but your body's needs have not. Your body, your vehicle, still needs fresh fruits, vegetables, lean protein and complex carbohydrates to function properly.

Just because your body is functioning, that doesn't mean it's healthy or that it's functioning at capacity. Picture your car. How does it run? Is it a smooth-running machine like a BMW, or are you getting around in an old jalopy? Both of them get you from Point A to Point B, but let's face it, which one is a more comfortable and more reliable ride?

Picture your body. How does it run? Is your body fit and active? Could you climb over a log or swim across a river if you had to? Or is your body inactive and unfit? Do you sometimes breathe heavily doing daily activities? Both types of bodies are a reality in our world today.

When I was a Peace Corps Volunteer, I lived in Côte d'Ivoire, West Africa for two years. During that time, I learned and experienced a great deal. While there, I read a compelling book by a fellow volunteer from another African country (I apologize, but I can't remember the name of the author or book). In it, the author told a story about arriving in her assigned village and being received by a greeting in the local dialect which translated to "are you in your skin today?" The author said that at first she didn't understand what they meant. Then finally, through different avenues and months of trial and error, she began to understand the villagers just meant essentially 'are you comfortable today?'

Are you "in your skin?" Are you comfortable where you are, with what your body can do for you? Are you confident you're treating your body respectfully? That is, how it would want to be treated? By *treated*, I mean physically, emotionally, spiritually, nutritionally, medically, psychologically, physiologically.

If you aren't completely comfortable in your body, then it's time to evaluate yourself and ask your body what it needs from you. Sit with your body, your vehicle: feel it, hug it, love it, and allow it to tell you what it needs. Offer it natural food choices and "listen" to your body. Sometimes it'll need something that's not a 'natural food' choice, and that's okay. Sometimes my body screams at me that it wants a hamburger, fries and, yes, a soda pop. I especially crave this trio the morning after drinking a few too many beers! I don't make a habit of drinking too much alcohol, but it makes me feel good for awhile. However, ultimately it doesn't make my body, my vehicle, run at top performance and I know it. I don't overdo drinking alcohol because I know better, and if I did it too often, I recognize it wouldn't make me feel good long-term. I know precisely how my body works, and I appreciate it for what it does for me, so I want to give it what it deserves. It deserves a little bit of a lot of different things, including lots of fresh fruits and vegetables, complex carbohydrates, and lean protein (beans, seeds, nuts, and the occasional animal sources).

Of course, there so many reasons we make any choice. We all have a Family of Origin (FOO) and Culture of Origin (COO) that shape and form who we are. We each have a personal story, background, and history. Many of us have suffered some form of trauma in our lives. Some of us had such horrific things happen to us that we'd like as few people as possible to know about them. Some of these experiences create negative images of ourselves in our heads, and we cope as best we can.

We have to adapt to our surroundings, we have to move on no matter what terrible deeds have been done to us. We are here and here we will stay until our lives are over. There are things you can do to feel better. Some of them might include psychotherapy, physical therapy, nutritional therapy, medical treatment, chiropractic or other natural medicine choices. I don't know what anyone else needs in order to be in his or her skin, I only know about myself. I know what goes on inside my skin. And I know there are things I can do to help my body run at maximum performance and endurance. I also know there are things I can do that aren't the best for me. I want to help you make informed choices.

There are so many things we can't control, but we can control what we eat. It's one of the first things we learn intrinsically (from within your own body): we learn how to suck our mother's breast, or the nipple of a bottle. Later, we learn that we can feed ourselves and sometimes mommy and daddy don't like what we feed ourselves, but they can't do a thing about it. That may run over into other areas of our lives, such as with boyfriends, girlfriends, spouses, etc.

Feeding ourselves is one thing over which we have complete control. That wasn't always the case for humans. Before the last 100 years, we relied on our neighbors, family, friends, clan members, and tribes to hunt and gather, plant and plow, etc. But, now, it's all on us: we're solely responsible for choosing for ourselves and our families. Unfortunately we don't always accept the best information about what to choose, or consider the best choices available to us.

In the last 50 (or fewer) years, we humans (namely Americans, but sadly, now much of the rest of the world as well) have actually been allowing companies to sell us products without even realizing it. Think about it, humans were eating foods found in nature for thousands and thousands of years. Then, bam! The Industrial Revolution arrived and humans drastically changed their diets and lifestyle practices in a relatively short time of about 100 years. Today, a few companies are making a lot of money off our current food supply. We receive media messages from businesses trying to unload high profit margin foods and we get confused. What are we supposed to do? Sometimes what we do is go out and purchase what is convenient, tasty and cheap, or simply what we see advertised.

There will always be access issues; many people do not have a choice about what's available to them. The University of Pennsylvania conducted a study that showed people living in neighborhoods dense with fast-food joints are more likely to be obese than people living in neighborhoods with full service restaurants. More fast-food means there are less fresh produce and whole grain choices available. I worked in an inner city area like this and the one grocery store had a very limited produce section. With fewer choices we must learn to control how much goes inside our bodies. It may require making more of your own meals at home, which actually saves money. It's cheaper, healthier and I think more fun to eat from your own kitchen, or at a friends' house.

I was once told by a mechanic that it didn't matter what fuel I put in my car, because it wasn't a high performance engine. He said that some engines were high performance and benefited from the better gasoline, but that I would be wasting my money buying the 'better' stuff. Not so for your body, your vehicle. Generally all humans' bodies run more efficiently with specific fuels (foods). Of course, there are different body types that run better on certain fuels than other types, and we'll explore that as well.

Remember, your body is a living thing, after all; it's not a trash can! Until very recently in the history of humanity, human beings basically had the same diet and medical treatment practices forever. Nowadays we're letting major corporations and people making a lot of money sell us what might not be the best for our health, but for their wealth. Isn't it time to get back to basics and back to nature – back to eating as nature intended, not as some conglomerate focused on making maximum profit tells us to do? Let's get back to the basics and eat real food again! Let's eat food that our bodies were created to eat. We're supposed to eat a real strawberry, not a corn syrup-based stick artificially flavored, colored, and twisted up to look and taste like one.

My Body, My Vehicle is simply a guide to learning about the human body's functions so that you can become your own mechanic. You're the closest one to your body; you probably know it better than anyone else. Now you can get to know your body even more. Here's a brief overview of what's inside the book.

Chapter Overview

In the following pages we'll explore our bodies and look at human nutrition and metabolism in a simple and easy-to-follow format. I think it's important for everyone to understand how their bodies work. Once you get to know the ins and outs of how your one of-a-kind, totally awesome machine works, you'll find it much easier to filter through all the information and products that confront you. It's time we invest in our bodies, our vehicles, and help them to run as smoothly and efficiently as possible.

Having visited more than 15 countries around the world, I am fortunate to have learned from many cultures through my travels, work experiences, and educational choices. In order to help me communicate the body's processes, I have taken the liberty to combine what I have learned from Western, Eastern and Traditional cultures.

In Chapter One, **Your Body is Your Vehicle**, we detail the nine systems of our body and focus on the digestive system. You will complete a frame assessment in order to determine which of the three frame types, or combination of types, you have. Each of us moves around in a particular type of frame, and knowing your frame will help you make the food and lifestyle choices that best suit your particular frame.

Every vehicle takes some kind of fuel, and Chapter Two, **Food is Fuel,** helps you to determine which fuel is best for your frame. It doesn't really matter what kind of fuel you put into most cars, the machine will run. It's the same with your body. However, I'll bet the Andretti brothers take great care in the kind of fuel they put into their race cars. And for the machine called your body, it likes nice, clean-running fuel for maximum efficiency.

In order to make the most of your machine, you have to know how to manage the market place. So, in Chapter Three, we'll walk through **Supermarket Savvy**, navigate the aisles of your average supermarket, read labels, and learn other tricks of the trade. We'll also take you into a Health Food Store and compare prices and products, because you might as well shop around for the best fuel at the best price, right?

That brings us to Chapter Four, **Media Madness**. If the Department of Health and Human Services, together with the National Institute of Health, has spent significant tax dollars teaching youth how to uncover media messages, I think we all ought to learn about it, too. The bottom line is that those food marketers are thinking of their bottom line, not yours (pun intended).

Chapter Five is **Movement Matters**. You guessed it: you have to take that vehicle of yours for a daily test drive! It's easier than you think to get those crucial 30 minutes of movement in every day.

Now that you're ready to make the right choices to keep your machine running at top performance, you need a plan to put it into action. So, Chapter Six is **The Road Map** which gives pointers on how to get on the highway to health and stay there. In order to make the right choices, you have to know what works, so we'll take the positive approach and look at everything you like about the current state of your body and its health. We also have some other tools and helpful hints to help keep you cruising on the highway to health throughout life.

Start Your Engines!

Chapter One

Your Body IS Your Vehicle

Your body is a wonderland ~ John Mayer

My Body, My Vehicle

Do you take care of your car? Do you give it tune-ups and oil changes so it runs smoothly? Do you keep the tires at a good air pressure to get better gas mileage? Do you periodically take it for a test drive to keep the battery charged?

Do you take care of your body? Do you nourish it by eating healthy meals with reasonable portion sizes? Do you drink plenty of water throughout the day? Do you breathe deeply and soundly to clear your exhaust pipes? Do you take your body for a daily test drive?

Your body is a vehicle: it functions like any other piece of machinery and it needs to be treated with care and respect. It is the one thing that is going to carry you around for your entire life, and it's worth the effort to learn how it works, so you're able to give it what it needs. Learning how your body works and giving it what it needs to run efficiently is like buying a lifetime warranty.

You don't have to take a lesson in anatomy and physiology to understand the basics of the human body. However, I believe it's important to learn the basics in order to get the full picture of how to get the most of your body as your vehicle. Many people know more about their car than they do about their insides. It's time to take control of your body in a new way and develop a new relationship with it.

Your Body, Your Vehicle

Think of your body as a vehicle. What is the shape of the vehicle you cruise around in? If your body was a vehicle, what would it be? Would it be a Ferrari, a Jeep, a Prius or one of a kind?

Draw a sketch on paper or in your mind's eye of your vehicle; think about it as you coast through this book. The image you come up with now may change. Perhaps today you're a Hummer and in a few months, after you've had time to reflect and make some changes, you may see yourself as a Corvette. One of the beautiful things about our bodies is that they are very receptive to change and they are very adaptable.

If you were a part of a car, what would you be? Are you the gear shift, a multi-tasker who's always changing gears? Are you the fuel system? Do you keep things running at full speed? Or, are you the passenger seat, laid back and enjoying the ride? All of these parts of the car help make it what it is: a functioning machine that gets you places. Just like your body.

Nine Body Systems

Our bodies are so similar to a vehicle that we even have just about the same number of systems. A car has eight systems and the human body is made up of nine systems. The car's systems are the Brake System, Engine, Cooling System, Heating & A/C, Electrical System, Steering and Suspension, Emission System, and Transmission. Similarly, the body's systems are the Circulatory, Digestive, Endocrine, Excretory, Immune, Muscular, Nervous, Respiratory, and Skeletal. All these systems work together to make up our beautiful bodies which *are wonderlands.*

The body systems work together in a most fascinating way; the body is truly not only an incredible machine, but I think it's the most beautiful work of art that has ever been created!

---

1. The Circulatory System can be looked at as the life pump. **The heart** is responsible for this system. The heart consists of a group of hollow chambers and each one acts as a little pump that circulates blood throughout the body to keep us alive. Arteries carry blood away from the heart, and veins carry blood back to the heart, working together in a rhythmic cycle. Red blood cells carry oxygen from the lungs to the rest of the body, and white blood cells protect the body from infection. *See Immune System.*

2. The Endocrine System is a little-known arrangement with a big job. Its duties are so diverse; it's tough to do it justice in a few sentences. The endocrine system is made up of a handful of glands that control, regulate, and coordinate many of the other systems. The most amazing part of this system is that it does it all through chemicals called *hormones.* The **thyroid, parathyroid, pituitary, thymus, pancreas, and adrenal** glands, along with some organs, such as **kidneys and stomach,** produce the hormones that take part in digestion, metabolism and reproduction, they regulate feelings of hunger or fullness, fatigue, and body temperature.

3. The Excretory System: You can probably guess what this system does. Yep, it gets rid of unwanted materials, otherwise known as *waste,* from our body. Our body produces waste that we must eliminate or it can become toxic to us. But our bodies are so efficient we have organs and glands that move the waste right out of it. The organs that mostly deal with this system are the **lungs and kidneys**. The lungs get rid of water vapors and carbon dioxide (air), the kidneys help excrete typical solid waste like urine and stool. Sweat glands help get rid of salts.

Unfortunately, sometimes we eat man-made, chemically processed, products that our systems don't know how to remove and that's when we can develop disease.

4. The Immune System is your body's defense mechanism. The immune system is what responds to stress, injuries and viruses. The general immune response is to an injury, bacteria, or virus which invades your body. What happens next is a series of occurrences of non-specific reactions, like inflammation, redness, or swelling. Your body produces **free radicals**, which act as little attack warriors that kill the invaders with rapid fire. However, they can also attack healthy cells if those get in the way.

When our bodies don't need the free radicals anymore, they stand by. Certain **vitamins** are responsible for firing the free radicals. As the immune response continues, it gets more complicated. White blood cells and immune tissues (a.k.a. lymphocytes), produce proteins called antibodies that kill the intruders and leave other cells undamaged. Miraculously, our body stores and remembers the recipe for each antibody it created to destroy specific intruders, which makes for a quicker immune response to a similar intrusion in the future.

5. The Muscular System is our movement megastore; this is the vehicle, the hot rod, your dream machine! Without muscles we couldn't do anything: not eat, laugh, sing, dance, blink, smile, or breathe! About 40% of a man's and 25% of a woman's body weight is muscle. This is the body's most abundant tissue and plays an important in role in our daily lives.

There are more than **600 muscles** that move us across this beautiful planet. The odd thing is they pull, not push; they move (contract) and relax. We can push because there are so many muscles pulling in different directions. Muscles are bundles of cells and fibers attached to the bones by tendons and other tissues and are linked to the brain by the **nervous system**.

The tiny cells of our muscles use chemical energy from the food we eat to make us move. Without food, and certain nutrients, like protein, your muscles wouldn't be able to make the energy they need to contract!

There are three types of muscles; Cardiac, Smooth, and Skeletal
  ➢ **Cardiac muscles** are only in the heart, and they power the movements that pump blood through the body.
  ➢ **Smooth muscles** cover the internal organs, such as the liver and stomach. Both cardiac and smooth muscles are called **involuntary** muscles because they cannot be controlled willfully.
  ➢ **Skeletal muscles** are **voluntary** muscles, so we can tell them what to do. These are the ones that hurt after a big workout.

6. The Nervous System is our control center, and that's why it's also called the Central Nervous System. It contains the **brain and spinal cord**. The nervous system receives input from our senses through neurons, or nerve cells. This is how we see, hear, smell, touch and feel, among other things.

7. The Skeletal System, or bone zone as it's sometimes called, is made up of, yes, **bones**. Our muscles attach to **bones** in order to give our bodies structure, which allows us to move. Not all bones are joined by muscles; some are joined by flexible parts called **joints**, which give them more elasticity, because, remember, muscles only pull. Besides giving us the ability to stand tall, our bones also make blood cells and store useful minerals, like calcium.

> **The smallest bones in our bodies are in our ears and the body's largest bone is the thigh bone, or femur.**

8. Respiratory System, or airbags, allows us to breath in oxygen, which is vital for life. All the cells in our bodies need **oxygen**. The body gets oxygen from the air that we breathe in through the nose. This air then travels a long way through the wind pipes and voice box to get to our lungs. Rib muscles contract to pull ribs up and out. The diaphragm muscle contracts to pull down the lung tissues, which expand to suck in air. Next, we breathe out through our mouth to get rid of the gasses that the body doesn't need. In doing so, the rib muscles relax, the diaphragm muscle relaxes, and lung tissues return to a resting state, which forces air out. Voila! You're alive and breathing!

We take more than 17,000 breaths every day! Breathing is such an important part of our daily lives, yet many of us don't even realize we're doing it. Many people aren't actually breathing correctly, their breaths are too short and not deep (or penetrating) enough. Studies show that deep breathing can reduce stress and stress related disorders, such as panic attacks, depression and digestive problems. Some studies even indicate deep breathing techniques have cured certain types of cancer. For this daily, usually mindless, activity, it's good practice to be more mindful of your breaths.

> **Breathe deeply through your nose as much as you can to fill your lungs, and then release the breath through your mouth. Do this as many times as you can, whenever you think about it.**

9. The Digestive System
When you think of digestion, you might conjure up thoughts of metabolism and what we eat. Digestion is what your body does to break down the food you eat, so that it can be absorbed throughout the nine systems and give you the energy you need to go places. It is one of your body's most important tasks! Your digestive system is like your car's filter system.

Why is the digestive system so important?
The food we eat is not in a form that the body can digest, or use as nourishment. Digestion is the process in which the food and drink we take in is broken down into smaller parts so that the body can use them to build and nourish cells and give us energy.

How is food digested?
Most medical philosophies throughout the world view digestion as a long process that mixes our food, moves it through the digestive tract, and breaks down the large pieces of food into smaller pieces (more specifically, molecules). Those molecules have duties and tasks that they perform, which we'll get into in the next chapter.

Most people might think digestion begins in the mouth, when we chew and swallow, and finishes in the anus with excretion. That is partially correct, but digestion actually begins even before we take the first bite of food. The smell of the food (and even the thought of it) gets digestive juices (saliva) flowing in the mouth. Once past the mouth, the smaller bits of food enter the large, hollow organs of the digestive system. These organs have muscles that allow their walls to move. This movement of the organ walls propels food and liquid and also shakes it up. The muscles of the organs push the food through the system like waves rolling along the shore. These muscles are so strong that they can push food through the digestive system even while you're upside down, although that is not recommended!

One digestive philosophy is that cold drinks (straight from the fridge or iced) can put out one's "digestive fire," causing the whole digestive process to slow down.

The digestive system is a series of hollow organs joined in a long, twisting tube from the mouth to the anus. Inside this tube is a lining called the *mucosa*. In the mouth, stomach, and small intestine, the *mucosa* contains tiny glands that produce juices to help us digest (break down) food.

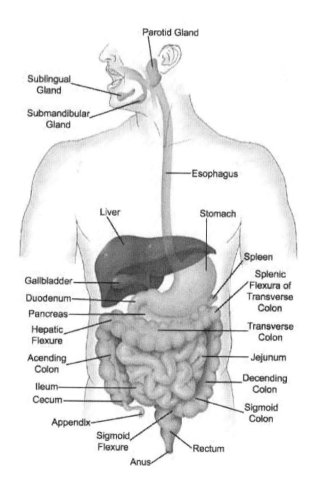

* I borrowed the above diagram from the web at
http://4pack.files.wordpress.com/2009/06/digestion-process2.jpg
It's far better than anything I could create on my own...

The Six Steps of Digestion:

1. Food begins its digestion in the mouth, where saliva activates some enzymes to help break it down into smaller particles:
   - Proteins get broken into amino acids
   - Fats get broken into fatty acids
   - Carbohydrates break down into simple sugars e.g., glucose, our body's most important fuel.

Saliva Glands:
   o **Parotid glands** are in the cheeks, right under the earlobes. Salty and bitter foods cause these glands to excrete *amylase*, the most potent saliva. *Amylase* starts to break carbohydrates into sugar, and this is why you can actually taste the food getting sweeter as you chew it.
   o **Submandibular glands** are in the back of the mouth beside each side of your lower jawbones and deep below the tongue. Sour and fatty foods activate these glands, which produce thick saliva that helps us swallow bulky foods.
   o **Sublingual glands** are just beneath the tongue, on the tissue floor of your mouth. Their thin saliva dilutes sugar and is triggered by sweet food and natural sugars in fruits and vegetables.

2. Swallowed food gets pushed past the esophagus, which connects to the throat above the stomach. At the intersection between the esophagus and stomach, there is a ring-like valve which closes the passage between the two organs. As the food approaches the closed ring, the surrounding muscles relax and allow the food to pass.

3. The food then enters the stomach, which has three jobs to do.
   a) The stomach must store the swallowed food and liquid. This requires the muscle of the upper part of the stomach to relax and accept large amounts of swallowed material.

> **You may have been told to chew your food slowly. This is so that your stomach can plan ahead and start making the enzymes needed to breakdown the food it recognizes.**

b) Next, the food, liquid, and digestive juices are mixed up. The stomach produces acid and an enzyme (pepsin) that digests protein to help it mix up and break down the food into even smaller molecules.

c) Finally, the stomach empties its contents slowly into the small intestine.

4. As the food is digested in the small intestine and dissolved into the juices from the pancreas, liver, and intestine, the contents are mixed and pushed forward to allow further digestion.

5. Finally, all of the digested nutrients are absorbed through the intestinal walls. Two other organs assist in the digestive process:

-   The **pancreas** produces many enzymes that help break down carbohydrates, fat and protein. The waste products of this process include undigested parts of the food, known as fiber, and older cells that have been shed from the *mucosa*.

-   These materials are propelled into the **colon**, where they remain, usually for a day or two, until the feces are expelled by a bowel movement. One of the digestive juices assisting in this process is bile, which is produced by the liver and stored in the gallbladder.

6. Now that the enzymes have helped break down the foods we've eaten into amino acids, fatty acids, or glucose, they can be used by the body for energy. These smaller molecules are absorbed in the *mucosa* and then passed into the bloodstream, where they are carried to cells throughout the body. After they enter the cells, other enzymes act to speed up or regulate the chemical reactions involved with "metabolizing" the compounds. During these processes, the energy from the compounds can be released and used by the body or stored in body tissues, especially the liver, muscles, and body fat.

Ever wonder why you start to feel hungry around five or six hours after your last meal? If it takes one hour for each of the six stages of digestion, that would equal six hours. That makes sense! Some of us, including me, tend to eat smaller, more frequent meals, in which case the digestive process might be a little speedier.

That's the digestive system for you! It is certainly not the complete story, as there are also a group of nerves and hormones that play huge roles in the digestive process. But since this is not a textbook, we'll skip all the gory details.

If you were one of the nine body systems, which one would you be?

Metabolism

Metabolism is a complex chemical process. It isn't necessary for every day living to be aware of the minute details, so it's easier to just think of it very simply as the process which controls how easily our bodies gain or lose weight. The process of metabolism is like a balancing act, with two activities happening at the same time:

1) The building up of body tissues and energy stores and
2) The breaking down of body tissues and energy stores to generate more fuel for body functions.

There are two types of metabolism:

Anabolism or **constructive metabolism** is the building up and storing component, and it:
- Supports the growth of new cells
- Maintains body tissues
- Stores energy for future use

During anabolism, small molecules are changed into larger, more complex molecules of carbohydrate, protein, and fat.

Catabolism or **destructive metabolism** is the process that produces the energy required for all cellular activity.
- This is where cells break down large molecules (mostly carbohydrates and fats) into glucose to release energy.
- This energy release provides fuel for anabolism, heats the body, and allows our muscles to contract and move our bodies.

As compounds are broken down into simpler substances, the waste products released through catabolism are removed from the body through the skin, kidneys, lungs, and intestines.

Many of the hormones of the endocrine system are involved in controlling the rate and direction of metabolism. The thyroid gland produces many hormones that regulate the body's energy as well as metabolism. Thyroxine, a hormone produced and released by the thyroid gland, plays a big role in determining how fast or slow the chemical reactions of metabolism continue in a person's body. Many people complain of hyper or hypo thyroid or other thyroid disorders for causing weight gain. That can happen, however it may be an excuse, as either condition is a serious one, and quite rare. If you think you may have a thyroid condition, please see your doctor as the condition can exacerbate if left untreated. The incidences of these diseases are on the rise and maybe a cause of food intolerances, commonly gluten (see information on food intolerances in the next chapter).

Lesser known facts:

- Some people burn calories at a slower rate than others.

- The more weight you carry, the *faster* your metabolism is likely running. The extra weight causes your body to work harder just to sustain itself at rest, so in many cases, the metabolism is always running a bit faster.

- There's a reason it's almost always easier to lose weight at the start of a diet, and harder later on. When you are very overweight your metabolism is already running so high that any small cut in calories will result in an immediate loss. Then, when you lose significant amounts of body fat and muscle, your body needs fewer calories to sustain it. That helps explain why it's so easy to regain weight after you've lost it.

    o If two people both weigh 250 pounds, and one got there by dieting down from 350 pounds, while the other one was always at 250, the one who got there by cutting calories is going to have a slower metabolism. That means they will require fewer calories to maintain their weight than the person who never went beyond 250 pounds.

How can you boost your metabolism?

- Exercise is the best. This includes aerobic workouts to burn more calories in the short term, and weight training to build the muscles that will boost your metabolism in the long run. Since muscle burns more calories than fat -- even while at rest -- the more muscles you have, the higher your resting metabolic rate, which means the more calories your body will be burning just to sustain you. Every pound of muscle in our body burns 35 calories a day, while each pound of fat burns just 2 calories per day.

- While 30 minutes of aerobic exercise may burn more calories than 30 minutes of weight training, in the hours post workout, the weight training has a longer-lasting effect on boosting metabolism. Having extra muscle also means you can eat more and gain less.

- Exercise while dieting is encouraged to burn calories, in addition, the exercise builds muscle and that what will help you burn more calories to maintain the weight loss.

- Is there a magic metabolism-boosting food? No. Any food will increase your metabolism, mostly in the first hour after you eat: that's when your system is most revved up.

- Protein generally requires about 25% more energy to digest. So, at least theoretically, a high-protein snack might speed up metabolism a little more than a carbohydrate-heavy food having the same number of calories.

- Your best bet for keeping metabolism revved up is to build muscles, snack on low-calorie, high-protein foods, and keep moving!

Metabolism Tips:

- ✓ Combine quality proteins, complex carbohydrates and healthy fats at every meal and snack
- ✓ Eat at least every four hours
- ✓ Control portions and calories
- ✓ Balance macronutrients with a ratio of 40 percent carbohydrates, 30 percent protein, and 30 percent fat, adjusting as needed
- ✓ Do not eat carbohydrates late in the day
- ✓ Do not eat in the 2 to 3 hours before going to bed
- ✓ Eat first thing in the morning (or within an hour of waking up)
- ✓ Eat whole, minimally processed foods
- ✓ Reduce intake of starchy vegetables, dried and canned fruits, excess soy, excess alcohol, full-fat dairy, fatty meats, canned foods, and caffeine

Metabolic Fuels

Metabolic fuel is another term for your total intake of food. Today, many health professionals aren't focusing as much on calories, because counting calories can be a confusing and cumbersome process. A calorie is a unit that measures how much energy a specified portion of food provides to the body. A candy bar has more calories than a banana, so it provides the body with more energy, and that's not always a good thing. Just as a car stores gas in the gas tank until it is needed to fuel the engine, the body stores calories primarily as fat. If you overfill a car's gas tank, it spills over onto the pavement. Similarly, if a person eats too many calories, they "spill over" in the form of excess fat on the body. Life threatening diseases occur when too much fat gets stored in our vital organs.

In order for the calories you consume not to be stored as fat, they must be burned off. If the amount of metabolic fuels you eat equals the amount of energy you expend, then your body is in a state of energy balance.

Your body goes through periods of fed states and fasting states over several days.
- Fed states are when your body is storing what it needs in the proper tissues and organs.
- Fasting states are when these reserves are being utilized by the body.

If your body has equal amounts of fed states and fasting states, it is in a state of energy balance, and over a couple of days, you won't gain any weight. On the other hand, if you take in more metabolic fuels than your body expends, you will spend more time in the fed state than in the fasting state. That means your body will build up more reserves than it uses, which means an increase in weight and body size. This increase in weight has some very serious health consequences!

> The way our bodies' digest and metabolize food is similar to a potbelly stove; they are both fires that burn fuel for energy, one burns wood, and the other burns food. If you want to heat your home with the stove, you fill it with logs; your body is the same. The stove usually doesn't get any wood at night but the cinders smolder and in the morning you stoke it with lots of wood to get it going through the day. Your system is the same, at night we don't feed our system, but in the morning, it requires a good balanced meal to burn nicely throughout the day (more details about this in Chapter 6).

Diabetes

The pancreas secretes hormones that help the body decide whether its main metabolic activity at a given time will be anabolic or catabolic. After eating a meal, usually more anabolic activity occurs because eating increases the blood glucose level and glucose is the main energy source for our cells. The pancreas knows the glucose levels have increased and releases the hormone insulin, which in turn signals cells to boost their anabolic activities. In other words, the released insulin tells the cells in our body to absorb the glucose and use it for energy. When the body has a hard time dealing with the glucose, it is called *diabetes*. There are two types of diabetes.

Type 1: Diabetes Mellitus occurs when the pancreas doesn't produce and secrete enough insulin. Symptoms of this disease include excessive thirst and urination, hunger, and weight loss. Some signs of diabetes may be bleeding gums, tingling feet or darkened skin patches on underarms and the neck. Long term, the disease can cause kidney problems, pain due to nerve damage, blindness, and heart and blood vessel disease. People with Type 1 diabetes need to receive regular injections of insulin to control blood sugar levels and reduce the risk of developing other serious health problems from diabetes. People with this disease either are born with it, or it develops in early childhood.

Type 2 Diabetes develops when the body can't respond normally to insulin. The signs and symptoms of this disorder are similar to those of Type 1 diabetes. Type 2 diabetes used to be called *Adult Onset Diabetes* because it occurred only in overweight, sedentary (inactive) adults. Today, many children and teenagers are developing this disorder so the medical profession has to use its scientific name, Type 2 Diabetes. Overweight and lack of physical activity is thought to play a major role in the body's decreased responsiveness to insulin. Controlling blood sugar levels reduces the risk of developing the same kinds of long-term health problems that occur with Type 1 Diabetes.

Diabetes is a major health concern in the United States. Each year there are 1.6 million new cases of diabetes most of which are Type 2. People who have diabetes incur two times the amount of medical costs than those without the disease. Diabetes costs our health care system roughly $174 billion a year. As we get older, we can all be at risk for developing Type 2 Diabetes because our bodies start to produce less insulin. Children should not have to suffer this condition and today, they do! Good ways to prevent changes in your blood sugar are simply living a healthy life with plenty of regular exercise, and eating a healthy, well balanced diet.

Body Mass Index (BMI)

Body mass index (BMI) is a measure of body fat based on height and weight that applies to adult men and women. BMI is the standard indicator of total body fat, or the proportion of bodyweight that is fat. The amount of total body fat a person has is related to his or her risk for serious diseases and even death. When a person has too much fat, they are at risk for becoming obese and are susceptible to the diseases associated to it.

Some of the major causes of death linked to obesity are:
- Cancer (breast, prostate and colorectal)
- Atherosclerosis
- Coronary heart disease
- High Blood Pressure
- Stroke
- Respiratory diseases

BMI Categories:

Desired range (low risk) = 20 – 25
Overweight (moderate risk) = 25 – 30
Obese (high risk) = 30 – 35
Morbidly obese = > 40

BMI scores below 18.5 are related to under-nutrition.

To calculate your BMI:
Body Mass Index is calculated by your weight in kilograms divided by your height squared (in meters). BMI = weight (kg)/height^2 (m).

For example, my if my weight is 115 lbs or 52 kg (1 lb = .45 kg) and my height is 5 feet 2 ½ or 1.6 meters (1 foot = .30 meters). That translates to 52/2.56 so my BMI is 20. I am within the desired range and not at risk for weight related diseases. **If you're having difficulty figuring out the formula, there are websites online that will do the math for you. If you have access to a computer, run a search for Body Mass Index formula.*

Body Mass Index (or BMI score) has some limitations.

BMI Limitations are:
- It may **overestimate** body fat in athletes and others who have a muscular build.
- It may **underestimate** body fat in older persons and others who have lost muscle mass.

Though this is not a perfect science and not a perfect determinant for how healthy you are or what percent of body fat you have, it is the most widely used measure today for obesity disease risk factors. For the majority of the population it is a fine measure. As the limitations indicate, if a person is very muscular they may have a BMI that puts them in the obese category, I'm sure no one would say that Will Smith or Tom Cruise are overweight or obese, but because they are so buff, their BMI's would say so. Chances are you and I don't have personal trainers and we don't work out four hours a day, so we probably don't need to worry that our BMI is misleading.

Basal Metabolic Rate (BMR):

The BMR, is a measure of the rate at which a person's body "burns" energy (calories) while at rest (not sleeping). The BMR can play a role in a person's tendency to gain weight. For example, a person with a low BMR (who burns fewer calories while at rest or sleeping) will tend to gain more pounds of body fat over time, compared with a similar-sized person with an average BMR who eats the same amount of food and gets the same amount of exercise.

BMR is calculated in controlled settings, so we won't be able to determine what your rate is in this book. The important thing to know is that there are many factors which affect the way your body burns up the food you eat, and, to some degree, it is inherited. Sometimes health problems can affect a person's BMR, which also decreases with age and loss of lean body mass (muscle). The good thing is a person can actually change their BMR.

Because BMR decreases with less lean body mass, exercising more will not only cause a person to burn more calories directly from the extra activity itself, but becoming more physically fit will increase BMR, as well. BMR is influenced by body composition - people with more muscle and less fat generally have higher BMRs.

Besides exercise, eating well makes a difference in BMR and how our bodies store fat. High fat meals take more time to go through the digestive process. That's why you may feel tired and sluggish after a high fat meal. This is because your body is taking more time and working harder to break down that meal and make it useful. Fat has 9 calories per gram, whereas the other macronutrients have 4 calories per gram, so it is harder to digest. This is another reason eating whole unprocessed nutritious foods are the right choice. Your body has a better chance to use the foods you eat with the least amount of effort when there are whole grains, plenty of fruits and vegetables and limited fat, meat and sugar for it to process.

Isn't the body an amazing and beautiful thing? For all it does for us, it doesn't ask a lot in return; only that we treat it well and feed it well. In Chapter Two, *Food Is Fuel,* we'll discuss how to properly feed it and many of the things that can happen when we don't.

We'll also take a look at the different parts (nutrients) that make up the food we eat and what components (molecules) they get broken down into for use by our bodies. After learning more about how your system runs, you should have enough information to make some great choices to keep your body running at maximum capacity.

Frame Assessment

Before we start learning more about the human body, take the following assessment to determine the type of **Frame** you have. You were born with your particular frame and it may not change that much, but according to your diet and lifestyle, it be can be altered. Most people are a combination of the different frames, or equal parts of two of them, but usually one predominates.

These frames are not meant to be stereotypes; they are to show typical bodily tendencies and to point out potential areas of excess. Put a check mark next to each item that relates to you. Count up the totals for each frame. The one you have the most marks for is your frame(s).

Sky   Total: _____

Bodily Structure

- [ ] Lean with little muscular definition, you may be very tall (man over 6 feet and woman over 5'8) or very short (man under 5'5 and woman under 5'3)
- [ ] Thin as a child
- [ ] Don't easily gain weight
- [ ] Rough, dry, darker-toned skin that easily chaps
- [ ] Curly, dry or dark hair
- [ ] Small, active dark brown, grey, or slate blue eyes
- [ ] Cold hands and feet

Bodily Tendencies

- [ ] Prefer warmer weather
- [ ] Low stamina and endurance, don't easily sweat
- [ ] Very active, but tire easily
- [ ] You don't need a lot of sleep and have disruptive sleep
- [ ] Thirst comes and goes, you like warm liquids
- [ ] Hunger is variable; sometimes you forget to eat, or your eyes are "bigger than your stomach"
- [ ] Like to snack and nibble
- [ ] Bowel movements are often hard and dry and you tend to get constipated

Bodily Disposition

- [ ] Short concentration span; you learn quickly and forget just as quickly
- [ ] Easily change your mind, difficulty making decisions
- [ ] Curious and restless
- [ ] Exercise helps you feel more mentally relaxed
- [ ] Can be nervous or anxious under stress
- [ ] Talkative
- [ ] Creative thinker, you don't care for routine

Sun   Total: _____

Bodily Structure

- [ ] Medium sized, well proportioned frame; moderately muscular.
- [ ] Medium as a child, may have gained and lost weight
- [ ] Easily gain and lose weight (if you put your mind to it)
- [ ] Oily, fair or soft skin, and you tend to have a lot of moles or freckles, acne prone
- [ ] Fine, silky hair, blond, red or brown; may grey or bald early
- [ ] Piercing, light green, grey, or amber eyes
- [ ] Skin is warm, hands and feet are usually warm

Bodily Tendencies

- [ ] Prefer cooler weather
- [ ] Moderately active and sweat easily
- [ ] Like to move and get physical, enjoy competitive sports
- [ ] Sleep soundly and don't require a lot of sleep
- [ ] Usually thirsty and enjoy cold drinks
- [ ] Good appetite, may get irritable if you miss a meal or can't eat when hungry
- [ ] Likes chicken, eggs, fish, beans and other high protein foods
- [ ] Loose, regular bowel movements, at least once or twice a day

Bodily Disposition

- [ ] Good short and long term memory
- [ ] Like to share opinions, make decisions rapidly
- [ ] Tendency towards jealousy
- [ ] Exercise helps you control emotions
- [ ] Can be aggressive and easily angered under stress
- [ ] Ambitious, smart and like to lead
- [ ] Organized thinker, like routine (especially if you create it)

Moon

Total: _____

Bodily Structure

- [ ] Thick, large frame
- [ ] Plump in childhood
- [ ] Gain weight easily, harder to lose
- [ ] Pale, thick, oily skin
- [ ] Thick, wavy hair, may be light or dark in color
- [ ] Dark (black or blue), large eyes with thick lashes
- [ ] Skin is cool to the touch, but you are not cold

Bodily Tendencies

- [ ] Like all weather, but prefer it warm
- [ ] Strong endurance and stamina
- [ ] Prefer leisurely activities best
- [ ] Sleep deeply and a lot
- [ ] Not excessively thirsty
- [ ] Good appetite and you like to eat: you can skip a meal, but would rather not
- [ ] Love breads and fatty, starchy foods
- [ ] Slow, heavy, regular, and daily bowel movements

Bodily Disposition

- [ ] Learn slowly and you have a great memory
- [ ] Slow to make a decision, but stick to it
- [ ] Loyal with a tendency toward possessiveness
- [ ] Exercise helps you control your weight that diet alone can't
- [ ] Tend to avoid difficult situations
- [ ] Calm and tolerant
- [ ] Like to follow a plan, routine works well for you

More about Sky, Sun, Moon

The information on Sky, Sun and Moon (not their real names) is based on an ancient medicine that's still practiced in India (and around the world) today. Called Ayurveda (*I-yer- veda*), this is the world's oldest science and it means "Science of Life." It was developed in approximately the 8th century B.C. and is still appropriate, perhaps especially for today's society. Because we have so many choices available to us and so many diseases, this could be the one thing that saves us. I was certified in Ayurvedic Nutrition 15 years ago when I received my Bachelor of Science in Nutrition at Bastyr University in Seattle, WA and I continually take courses on the topic. I personally use the principles and share them with my clients. It is basically a diet and lifestyle practice, and I have helped some very ill clients reverse diseases by using these principals to make simple changes in their diets.

Many of the concepts can seem counterintuitive and the words are in Sanskrit, so it can be confusing and not easy to grasp. For the sake of ease in understanding and bringing this effective medicine to the general public, I have renamed the terms. This is not out of disrespect for the wise creators of the practice, but out of a realization that it may help my friends and family and those who read this book to understand the value of it and make it more easily accessible to Western ears. There is a great deal more information to know than what I am going to convey in these few pages. I want to clarify that am not an Ayurvedic doctor. That takes a full six-year medical program. But I am educated on the subject and have seen it work, so I am going to try to simplify its concepts for you. The contents in this book do not even touch the surface of all the amazing information available on the subject. What I provide is a very simple guide to understanding your body type, or frame and easy ways that you can help keep it healthy and in balance. For more information, look up Ayurvedic centers in your neighborhood, and check for resources online, in the back of this book, or at your library or bookstore.

Finding Balance

Situations in our lives can alter our frames and cause changes or imbalances in our frameworks. For instance, normally you may find that as a child you were always running around playing with the other kids in the neighborhood. You came inside only when your folks called you in. You were rail thin and ate every meal served to you. Then, you went away to college and started eating lots of pasta noodles and pizza because they were affordable and easy to fix. Added to that, you began eating chocolate chips or other sweets and before you knew it, you could finish an entire bag of cookies. Now, you find yourself overweight, sluggish, and don't like to play outside the way you did as a kid. Your Sky is out of balance and your Moon is too high, so you'd need to avoid sweet, warming foods and start eating drier, cooling Sky foods to bring your Sky back up.

Or, maybe as a child you were chubby, but got involved in ballet and started to put yourself on strict diets in order to maintain a certain weight. With that, you may have become anxious and unable to sleep well. This meant your frame was out of balance. Your Moon frame developed an imbalance in Sky, so now in order to feel balanced again you would work on balancing your Moon and Sky. In order to balance Moon again, you need to start eating cooked, calming and warming foods. There may be psychological issues at work in this situation, and these we won't discuss, but if you can relate to this, it might be helpful to see a therapist.

Using myself as an example, I first learned about my frame type 15 years ago. Then, I was a Sky with some Moon. I didn't have a lot of Sun tendencies at all. Currently, I'm going through a lot of stress; a divorce, moving, starting my own business, being a single mom, etc. I haven't been eating the best diet, and cravings for French fries and Buffalo wings have gotten the best of me. With all the anger and fiery emotions surrounding my divorce, the stress, and adding the spicy fried foods, I have a lot more Sun. I've found myself being much more irritable at little things and I have even developed some issues with eczema, which I'd never before had. So, I really need to work on balancing my frame and getting the excess Sun out of my Sky!

Sky

Sky types tend to be very short or very tall, they are usually thin and their limbs (hands, arms, legs, fingers, etc.) may seem out of proportion or too long for their frame. They tend to have coarse, dry hair and skin and cold hands and feet. They do not like cold environments.

They are light and airy and may have trouble gaining weight. They're quick and speedy, and have less endurance than other frames. They have quick bursts of energy and then get exhausted. They're talkative and have nervous tendencies. They have a lot of energy and are usually very creative, bright, adaptable and flexible. They prefer warm weather and warm, cooked foods.

Health problems for Sky types can include constipation, gas, weak digestion and slow memory. Because of the dryness, they may suffer from arthritis, and have weak joints that make cracking or popping sounds. They are prone to getting 'the chills.' When out of balance they may develop insomnia, anxiety, and stress-related nervous disorders.

Sky people should avoid gaseous foods that create more wind, like the crucifers (broccoli, kale, collards, and cauliflower). They should eat frequent small meals of easily digestible foods to balance their blood sugar. Cold aggravates Sky so they should avoid cold beverages and drink warm water and tea. Even ice cream is too cool for Sky, and they should avoid it especially in the cooler winter months.

Sun

Sun types tend to have medium to large frames. They have a medium build and can be muscular. They have mild strength and endurance. Suns have soft, rosy toned skin and nails; they may have lots of moles, skin tags and freckles, and may become gray or bald prematurely.

These people are intelligent, resourceful, passionate, energetic, and adventurous. They are very alert and active, strong-willed, brave, and quick to anger or become jealous. They have huge appetites and may say they are 'always hungry,' because their metabolism is strong they are able to eat a lot of food and not gain weight. They are very thirsty and need to drink lots of water. Possessing a hot frame, they do not like heat and tend to seek shade on a sunny summer day.

Health problems with Sun tend towards skin problems like eczema, skin inflammation, pimples, acne, skin cancer, and poor vision. They may also have digestive problems like heartburn, acid stomach and ulcers.

When out of balance they may become hostile. Alcohol does not work well with Sun, and although they may like it, it can cause liver problems.

Sun people have big appetites, so they should eat more often, but consume cooler foods and avoid hot, spicy, sour food. Even black pepper is too hot for this fiery frame. Sweet, bitter and astringent tastes are more appropriate for them.

Moon

Moon types tend to be large and are heavy or thick boned. They tend to have thick, oily hair and skin, and have large doe-like eyes. They are typically strong and slow with lots of stamina and are good at physical labor. They have strong immune systems, so they may be more resistant to colds and the flu.

They are thoughtful, intelligent, shy, calm and possessive. They may tend towards greed, envy and over-attachment. They may be frugal and hold onto possessions. They are generally very grounded, loving and forgiving. Moons are predisposed to gain weight and may sleep a lot. They don't like cold weather or cold foods, but can tolerate it because of their strength.

Health problems with Moons tend towards obesity and obesity-related diseases, such as diabetes. They can be lethargic and not want to exercise, even though they should and need to in order to keep their weight in check. Moons love sweets, breads, starches and milk, but that weighs them down and creates a lot of mucus, so they may tend to have hay fever, congestion, sinus, and respiratory problems.

Moon frames are balanced by light, warm foods such as ginger and black pepper. Cold, sweet, sour, heavy and astringent foods can aggravate them. They should avoid cold, sweet foods like refined sugar, refined carbohydrates (white rice, white bread), milk, butter, ice cream and bananas.

Detailing Your Frame

"*Yatha Pinde Tatha Brahmande*" in Sanskrit this translates to "*whatever is true in the universe is true in the body.*" This basically means we are made up of the same elements as the universe, or nature, so if we want to be healthy, we should follow Mother Nature. This is why it is so important to pay attention to what we eat, and why there is an entire science and medical practice dedicated to nourishing the body.

Whether you're predominately a Sky, Sun or Moon, you would do well to find out how your frame runs best. Each of our unique frames runs best on different kinds of fuels. Sure, you can fill up on some of the fuels that are in your *not-so -good list*, but don't make a habit of it. By the way, none of our frames run well on fried foods. Think of it as detailing your body frame. Your body could use a good detail job just as much as your car.

While most of us have two frames that dominate our constitutions, we are all made of all three frame types; we each have different ratios of the three. Because we have various degrees of all three frames, either one of them can get out of balance. Back to my condition -- I was predominately Sky and Moon most of my entire life, fast forward to the dawning of midlife for me and all of the emotional and situational changes that have taken place and now I'm predominately Sun and Sky, my Moon is very faint. By making better choices for my frame over the last month, I've noticed a big difference and my frame and mood is rebalancing.

Some of this will take trial and error, testing different methods and making your own combinations. We are all so different and unique in our own particular makeup. So many of us are from diversified cultural and ethnic backgrounds and we have our own unique personalities and our bodies do, too. Although we all have eyes, hair, nails, bones, organs, etc, each of these has its genetic code unique to the individual. So, experiment with your frame, discover to which different kinds of foods, herbs and spices your body reacts best. (In Chapter 2 we discuss more about the frames and what role they play in digestion).

Keep in mind that there are ways an Ayurvedic practitioner can help determine imbalances in your frame other than with a check list frame assessment like the one in this book. There are other bodily signs, for example, your pulse tells a lot about the state of your frame. For information, see a specialist in your area.

The following information is adapted from lectures by the illustrious Dr. Virender Sodhi, M.D, N.D. As always, if your doctor or nutritionist recommended that you not consume something on your list of foods, consult him/her before indulging.

Nutrition and the Frames

Sky

The Sky frame is airy; they should eat warm, moist and heavier foods to balance the light, dry and cool energy. They should slow down and focus on their food and not eat while doing a number of other things at the same time (including watching TV). They tend to do best with smaller, more frequent meals throughout the day.

Vegetables

Most	Moderate	Least
Avocados	Alfalfa	Broccoli
Beets	Artichoke	Brussels sprouts
Black olives	Bell pepper	Cabbage
Carrots	Cauliflower	Chicory
Cilantro	Celery	Lettuce
Cooked onions	Chard	Mushrooms
Radishes	Chilies	Onions (uncooked)
Seaweed	Corn	Popcorn
Sweet potatoes	Eggplant	
Yams	Mustard greens	
	Okra	
	Potatoes	
	Spinach	
	Squash	
	Tomato	

Fruit

Most	Moderate	Least
Ripe banana	Apples	Unripe banana
Dates	Apricots	Cranberries
Figs	Oranges	Dried fruit
Grapefruit	Peaches	Unripe mango
Lemons/limes	Pears	
Ripe mango	Persimmons	
Papaya	Plums	
Pomegranate		
Raspberries		
Strawberries		

Grains

Most	Moderate	Least
Amaranth	Barley	Corn
Basmati rice	Buckwheat	Granola
Brown rice	Quinoa	
Couscous	Rye	
Oats		
Millet		
Wheat		

Beans

Most	Moderate	Least
Crushed lentils	Aduki beans	White beans
Mung beans	Chickpeas (garbanzos)	Whole lentils
	Kidney beans	Pinto beans
	Lima beans	Soy
	Tofu	Split peas

Seeds and Nuts

Most	Moderate	Least
Almonds	Coconut	Peanuts
Brazil nuts	Pistachios	
Cashews	Pumpkin seeds	
Flaxseed (ground)	Sunflower seeds	
Filberts	Walnuts	
Pecans		
Pine nuts		
Sesame seeds		

Dairy

Most	Moderate	Least
Butter	Cheese	Ice cream
Buttermilk		
Cottage cheese		
Ghee		
Milk		
Sour cream		
Yogurt		

Meats

Most	Moderate	Least
Eggs	Chicken	Beef
Fish	Lamb	pork
Shellfish	turkey	
Venison		

Oils

Most	Moderate	Least
Almond	Canola	Peanut
Butter	Coconut	
Flax	Mustard	
Ghee	Safflower	
Olive	Soy	
Sesame		

Sweeteners

Most	Moderate	Least
Agave syrup	Brown sugar	White sugar
Fructose		
Honey		
Maple syrup		
Molasses		
Raw sugar		
Stevia		
Sucanant (unrefined cane sugar)		

Spices

Most	Moderate	Least
Allspice	Black pepper	
Basil	Garlic	
Cardamom	Horseradish (wasabi)	
Cinnamon	Mint	
Cloves	Mustard	
Cumin	Saffron	
Fennel	Sea salt	
Fenugreek	Turmeric	
Ginger		
Nutmeg		

Sun

Sun's frame is fiery, so they should focus on cooling, slightly heavy, and mildly dry foods. They do well with three regular meals a day and snacks as needed.

Vegetables

Most	Moderate	Least
Alfalfa	Beets	Avocados
Asparagus	Carrots	Chilies
Black olives	Chard	Garlic
Brussels sprouts	Fresh corn	Tomatoes
Cabbage	Onions	Bell pepper
Cauliflower	Parsley	Eggplant
Cilantro	Potatoes	Tomato
Cucumbers	Radishes	
Green beans	Seaweed	
Lettuce	Spinach	
Mushrooms	Squash	
Okra	Sweet potatoes	
	Turnips	
	Watercress	
	Yams	

Fruit

Most	Moderate	Least
Apples	Apricots	Sour grapes
Bananas	Cherries	Grapefruit
Dates	Lemons/limes	Unripe fruit
Figs	Mangoes	
Grapes	Oranges	
Melons	Papaya	
Pears	Plums	
Persimmon	Raspberries	
Pineapple		
Pomegranate		
Prunes		

Grains

Most	Moderate	Least
Barley	Brown rice	Corn
Basmati rice	Buckwheat	
Couscous	Millet	
Granola	Rye	
Oats		
Quinoa		
Wheat (gluten can be a problem for our Sun friends)		

Beans

Most	Moderate	Least
Aduki	Chickpeas (garbanzos)	
Black beans	Kidney	
Black garbanzos	Lentils (whole)	
Lentils (crushed)	Split peas	
Lima	Soy	
Mung		
Tofu		

Seeds and Nuts

Most	Moderate	Least
Almonds	Pine nuts	Brazil nuts
Coconut	Pumpkin seeds	Cashews
Flaxseed (ground)	Sesame seeds	Filberts
Sunflower seeds	Cucumber seeds	Pecans
		Pistachios
		Walnuts

Dairy

Most	Moderate	Least
Buttermilk	Salted cheese	Sour cream
Cheese	Kefir	
Cottage Cheese		
Ice cream		
Milk		
Yogurt		

Meats

Most	Moderate	Least
	Chicken	Beef
	Eggs	Lamb
	Wild birds	Pork
	Fish	Shellfish

Oils

Most	Moderate	Least
Almond	Corn	Mustard
Butter	Sesame	Peanut
Coconut	Safflower	
Flax	Soy	
Ghee	Sunflower	
Olive		

Sweeteners

Most	Moderate	Least
Agave syrup	Brown sugar	White sugar
Brown rice syrup		
Fructose		
Honey		
Maple syrup		
Molasses		
Raw sugar		
Stevia		
Sucanant		

Spices

Most	Moderate	Least
Cardamom	Basil	Allspice
Cilantro	Cinnamon	Anise
Coriander	Cumin	Bay leaf
Fennel	Fresh Ginger	Black pepper
Fenugreek	Mint	Cloves
Saffron	Nutmeg	Dry Ginger
	Rock salt	Garlic
	Turmeric	Mustard
		Star Anise

Moon

The energy around a Moon's frame is slow, cool and heavy, so they need to counter that with warming, light, and dry foods. They require three meals a day and lunch should be the largest meal. They should make an effort to include a lot of variety in their diets, so as not to fall into a rut. They should be sure to get at least 30 to 60 minutes of some kind of physical activity every day.

Vegetables

Most	Moderate	Least
Alfalfa	Bell peppers	Cucumber
Asparagus	Cauliflower	Green olives
Beets	Corn	Potato
Broccoli	Eggplant	Sweet potato
Cabbage	Okra	Yams
Carrots	Parsley	
Celery	Peas	
Chard	Seaweed	
Chilies	Spinach	
Cilantro	Squash	
Green beans	Tomato	
Lettuce		
Mustard greens		
Turnip		
Watercress		

Fruit

Most	Moderate	Least
Apples	Papaya	Bananas
Blueberries	Pomegranate	Cherries
Cranberries	Prunes	Dates
Dried fruit		Figs
Lemon/lime		Grapefruit
Pineapple		Mangoes
Raspberries		Melons
Strawberries		Oranges
		Plums
		Tangerines

Grains

Most	Moderate	Least
Barley	Basmati rice	Couscous
Popcorn (air popped)	Brown rice	Oats (cooked)
Oats (dry)	Buckwheat	Wheat
Quinoa	Corn	White rice
	Millet	
	Rye	

Beans

Most	Moderate	Least
Aduki	Chickpeas (garbanzos)	
Black garbanzos	Kidney	
Lentils	Split peas	
Lima	Tofu	
Mung		

Seeds and Nuts

Most	Moderate	Least
Almonds	Coconut	Brazil nuts
	Pumpkin seeds	Cashews
	Sunflower	Filberts
		Pecans
		Pine nuts
		Sesame
		Walnuts
		Peanuts

Dairy

Most	Moderate	Least
Buttermilk	Fage	Butter
Soy milk	Goat milk	Cheese
	Kefir	Cottage cheese
		Ice cream
		Milk
		Sour cream
		Yogurt

Meats

Most	Moderate	Least
Chicken (poultry)		Beef
Fish (wild)		Eggs
Lobster		Lamb
Shrimp		Pork

Oils

Most	Moderate	Least
Flax	Coconut	Avocado
Mustard	Corn	Butter
Olive	Safflower	Ghee
Sesame	Soy	Peanut

Sweeteners

Most	Moderate	Least
Agave syrup	Honey	Brown sugar
	Sucanant	Fruit syrup
	Stevia	Maple syrup
		Molasses
		White sugar

Spices

Most	Moderate	Least
Allspice	Fennel	Salt
Basil	Nutmeg	
Black pepper	Saffron	
Cardamom	Turmeric	
Cayenne		
Cilantro		
Cloves		
Coriander		
Cumin		
Fenugreek		
Garlic		
Ginger		
Horseradish (wasabi)		
Mint		
Mustard		
Parsley		

NOTES

Chapter Two

Food is Fuel

Sugar is a type of bodily fuel, yes, but your body runs about as well on it as a car would. ~V.L. Allineare

Food is fuel, and we are lucky to be living in this time when we're able to enjoy a wide variety of metabolic fuels for our bodies. The dietary sources of our metabolic fuels are carbohydrates, fats, and protein. Alcohol is also a metabolic fuel, but we won't cover it in this book, since there is not a great deal of room for alcohol in a well-functioning body. The bottom line on alcohol is moderation; studies show a little alcohol may actually be good for digestion. One glass of red wine a day may be quite healthy, but that doesn't mean you should drink it daily and create and addiction. Occasionally is more like it.

If we have more metabolic fuel than our body can use, it is stored as fat, and one can become obese. Not enough fuel and one will be malnourished, which has a number of risk factors associated to it. Under nutrition is a problem, but it is not the basis of this book and we won't talk about the health problems related to it. The world at large is facing an **over** nourished epidemic. In other words, the world is becoming obese. It was estimated that in 2005, for the first time in human history, there were more overweight and obese people than underweight and hungry people on our planet! Although we are getting heavier, that doesn't necessarily translate to healthier. In fact, many obese people still suffer from under nutrition because they aren't getting the right amount of nutrients.

Nutrients

Nutrient *(noun):* a substance that must be consumed as part of the diet to give the body a source of energy for growth. Nutrients are substances that regulate bodily growth and energy production and are essential for normal body function.

Macronutrients

We need to consume all of the macronutrients every day. Some we need more of than others and there are many different theories on what ratios or percentages of each of them should make up our daily diet. The ratios I provide are an average guide to get your personal ratio see the suggestions in Chapter 6.

Carbohydrates (Carbs) 60% of total calories (range = 45% – 65%)
Carbohydrates = 4 grams per calorie.

Some of our most common foods contain mostly carbohydrates. Examples are bread, potatoes, legumes (beans, lentils and peas), rice, pasta, fruits, and vegetables. Many of these foods contain both starch and fiber. The digestible (useable) carbohydrates are broken down by enzymes in the saliva, in fluid produced by the pancreas, and in the lining of the small intestine.

There are two types of carbohydrates: complex and simple.

❖ **Simple Carbs (carbohydrates) = Starch**   This is digested in two steps:
   1. Enzymes (proteins that speed up biological functions) in the saliva and pancreas break down the starch into smaller molecules called *maltose*. Then, an enzyme in the lining of the small intestine splits the *maltose* into glucose molecules that can be absorbed into the blood.
   2. Glucose is carried through the bloodstream and used to provide energy for the body to function. What isn't used immediately is converted into glycogen in the liver and muscles where it is stored for later use.
      o Table sugar is another simple carbohydrate that must be digested to be useful. An enzyme in the lining of the small intestine digests table sugar into glucose and fructose, each of which can be absorbed from the intestinal lining into the blood.
      o Milk contains yet another type of sugar, lactose, which is changed into absorbable molecules by an enzyme called *lactase*, also found in the intestinal lining. Some people are lactose intolerant, which means their bodies don't produce enough *lactase* to digest dairy products.

o   Refined grains like white bread and pasta are also simple sugars. They rapidly convert to glucose in our system and aren't the healthiest choice, but okay once in a while.

❖ **Complex Carbs = Fiber** – 15% of carbohydrate calories. For women and children, try to get 20 grams, for men, 30 grams per day!

Fiber is a carbohydrate that the body can't digest. It is an important part of a healthy diet. It absorbs a lot of water so it helps form the bulk needed to create healthy bowel movements.

There are two types of fiber, soluble and insoluble, and they each have different functions and health benefits...

Soluble Fiber: It can dissolve in water and is eventually digested in the large intestine. It has limited bulk abilities. • Helps prevent blood sugar highs and lows • Lowers blood cholesterol • Lowers risk of heart disease • Helps control blood pressure	Insoluble Fiber : Does not dissolve in water and cannot be digested, so it helps speed stool transit. • Cleans bowel, binds toxins • Helps with regularity (preventing constipation) • Promotes better digestion • Lowers risk of bowel diseases
Oatmeal	Whole wheat products
Oat bran	Barley
Nuts and seeds	Couscous
Legumes	Brown rice
Beans	Bulgur
Dried peas	Whole grain breakfast cereals
Apples	Wheat bran
Pears	
Strawberries	
Blueberries	
Lentils	

Protein – 20% of total calories (range = 10% – 35%)
Protein = 4 grams per calorie

Foods such as meat, eggs, and beans have big molecules of protein that must be digested by enzymes before they can be used to build and repair body tissues.

An enzyme in the juice of the stomach starts the digestion of swallowed protein. Further digestion of the protein is completed in the small intestine. Here, several enzymes inside pancreatic juice and the lining of the intestine break down the bigger protein molecules into smaller molecules called *amino acids*. These small molecules can be absorbed from the hollow tubes of the small intestine into the blood and are then carried to all parts of the body to build the walls and other parts of cells, as well as our muscles and other tissues. When your body uses the protein you ingest to do its job, you have to replace it with more protein. Even adult bodies that are no longer growing require protein.

❖ **Amino Acids:** Our bodies need protein to rebuild muscles and other proteins, but more importantly, what it needs is the amino acids that make up the proteins in particular proportions. For adults there are nine essential amino acids: they are essential because our bodies cannot make them.

    o **The nine essential amino acids:**
- Histidine
- Isoleucine
- Leucine
- Lysine
- Methionine
- Phenylalanine
- Theronine
- Trypotophan
- Valine

❖ **Sources of Protein:** Because protein and the essential amino acids are found in the major dietary staples of most countries, It is highly unlikely that any adult will suffer from protein deficiencies. However, vegetarians and vegans who do not eat any animal protein may have a hard time getting enough protein. It is recommended that they eat high protein grains, such as quinoa and amaranth.

○   Meat, fish and eggs are generally viewed as rich animal sources of protein. Cereals, grains, nuts, and legumes are rich plant-based protein sources. The only grains that have insufficient protein are cassava (manioc), yams, corn and rice; anyone whose main staple comes from either of those grains will have to include small amounts of other protein sources, such as meat, fish, beans, legumes or nuts.

Fat – 20% of total calories (range = 20% – 35%)
Fat = 9 grams per calorie

Fat molecules are a rich source of energy for the body. Fat in the diet comes from butter and spreads, meat, fried foods and naturally occurring oils in nuts, seeds and some vegetables.

The first step in digestion of a fat, such as butter, is to dissolve it into the watery content of the intestinal cavity. The bile acids produced by the liver act as natural detergents to dissolve fat in water and allow the enzymes to break the large fat molecules into smaller molecules, some of which are fatty acids and cholesterol.

The bile acids combine with the fatty acids and cholesterol to help these molecules move into the cells of the mucosa. In these cells, the small molecules are formed back into large molecules, most of which pass into vessels (*called lymphatics*) near the intestine. These small vessels carry the reformed fat to the veins of the chest, and the blood carries the fat to storage depots in different parts of the body (otherwise known as saddlebags or love handles). (See chapter 3 for information about the different kinds of fats and other dietary sources).

Micronutrients

Vitamins

Another vital part of our food that is absorbed from the small intestine is the class of naturally occurring chemicals we call vitamins. They are also known as *micronutrients,* because the body needs a relatively small amount of them (along with coenzymes), because they work with enzymes to help regulate metabolism and release energy from food.

There are two different types of vitamins required by the body to function properly; they are classified by the fluid in which they can be dissolved:

- **Water-soluble vitamins** - all the B vitamins (B Complex) and vitamin C. These vitamins must be ingested daily, because they are not stored in the body and are excreted from the body within 4 to 24 hours.
- **Fat-soluble vitamins** - vitamins A, D, E and K. These can be stored in fatty tissue and the liver.

Vitamin A – Necessary for new cell growth and maintenance and repair of skin tissues and mucus membranes. Vitamin A aids in preventing night blindness, in fat storage, and as a protective antioxidant. The *carotenoids* are a type of vitamin A: the most popular *carotenoids* are *beta-carotene and lycopene,* both of which have been reported to help fight cancer.

Sources of vitamin A are green, yellow, or orange fruits and vegetables. Tomatoes have gotten a great deal of attention for having stores of lycopene, and livers (including fish liver oils) are animal sources.

Vitamin B Complex – This family of B vitamins maintain skin, eyes, hair, nerve and muscle health. They are also known as coenzymes, and help with enzyme reactions and energy production. Their vital role in nerve health is a reason they are often prescribed for stress reduction. The B vitamins work together, however, they are often broken down into their individual compounds. Below is a modified and abbreviated description of B Complex:

- Vitamin B1 (Thiamine) – Responsible for enhancing circulation, blood formation, carbohydrate metabolism and producing hydrochloric acid (vital part of digestion). This is another important protective antioxidant. Good sources of Thiamine are whole grains, like brown rice, wheat germ, rice bran, oatmeal, legumes, such as peanuts and peas, nuts, and dried fruits (raisins and prunes). Animal sources are egg yolks, fish, liver, pork, and poultry.

- Vitamin B2 (Riboflavin) – Important in the formation of red blood cells, producing antibodies, cellular respiration and growth, also oxygen use by hair, nails and skin. B2 is used in the treatment of cataracts, helps in metabolizing carbohydrates, fats and proteins. It is also needed for metabolizing the amino acid *tryptophan*, which converts to niacin in the body. Adequate amounts during pregnancy are needed (along with folate) to prevent damage to the fetus. Good sources of B2 include legumes, whole grains, egg yolks, dairy products (like milk, cheese and yogurt), fish, poultry, leafy green vegetables (spinach), avocados, and nuts.

- Vitamin B3 (Niacin & Niacinamide) – Another circulatory regulator and skin maintainer. It is useful in the function of the nervous system, metabolizing carbohydrates, fats, and proteins and producing hydrochloric acid. Good sources of Vitamin B3 are whole wheat products, wheat germ, brewer's yeast, corn flour, dairy products, eggs, fish, pork, broccoli, carrots, potatoes, and tomatoes.

- Vitamin B5 (Panothenic Acid) – The anti-stress vitamin, it helps in producing adrenal hormones and neurotransmitters, antibody formation, helps in energy production, and normal gastrointestinal tract functioning. Every cell in the body relies on this vitamin. Good sources are most fresh vegetables, legumes, mushrooms, whole wheat, brewer's yeast, nuts, eggs, pork, kidneys, livers, and saltwater fish.

- Vitamin B6 (Pyridoxine) – This mighty vitamin is involved in more body functions than almost any other nutrient. It plays a role in physical and mental health, and is necessary for producing hydrochloric acid and in fat and protein absorption. It is necessary for the nervous system and normal brain function. B6 is required to synthesize RNA and DNA, which are responsible for genetic coding. It activates many enzymes and plays a role in numerous other systems, including cancer immunity. Vitamin B6 can be found almost anywhere in food, with the highest quantities of this vitamin being in wheat germ, brewer's yeast, carrots, spinach, peas, sunflower seeds, walnuts, chicken, eggs, fish, and meat.

- Vitamin B12 (Cyanocobalamin) – Helps the body use iron, aiding in the prevention of anemia. B12 is necessary for digestion and food absorption, protein synthesis, and metabolizing carbs and protein. B12 aids in cell formation and longevity, prevents nerve damage, protects nerve endings, and assists memory and learning. Good sources of Vitamin B12 are found in dairy products, brewer's yeast, clams, eggs, kidney, liver, soy beans, seafood and sea vegetables such as, arame, dulse, hijiki, kelp, kombu, nori and wakame.

Vitamin C

Ah, the great antioxidant! Vitamin C is needed for more than 300 metabolic functions in our systems. Our bodies use it for tissue growth and repair, adrenal functions, healthy gums, anti-stress hormone production, and immune functions. It is crucial for collagen formation, and is also needed for iron absorption. It protects against and prevents cancer, helps lower cholesterol, lessens the effects of bruising and blood clotting, and so much more.

The body cannot make vitamin C, so it must be ingested. Being water soluble, much of the vitamin C we consume is lost in urine and that is why so many people take vitamin C supplements. Good dietary sources are berries, citrus fruits, and green vegetables.

Vitamin D

The "sunshine vitamin" acts like a vitamin and a hormone. It is needed for calcium and phosphorous absorption and utilization. Vitamin D is necessary for thyroid function, normal blood clotting, and growth and development of bones and teeth in children. It also protects muscles against weakness, and helps regulate heartbeat. Recently, much research has been done about vitamin D's ability to enhance immunity, and its usefulness in the prevention and treatment of many diseases, such as breast and colon cancers, osteoarthritis, osteoporosis, and multiple sclerosis. Some disorders associated to vitamin D deficiency are: autism, cancer (it destroys cancerous cells and prevents them from dividing), diabetes (Types 1 and 2), high blood pressure, rheumatoid arthritis, and seasonal affective disorder. Many people consume lots of vitamin C pills when they first feel symptoms of a cold, and now many people, including me, are starting to supplement with vitamin D as well, because of its immune enhancing functions.

Dietary sources of vitamin D are limited. Fatty fish, like salmon, is the best source. Next in line are dairy products, eggs, and some fortified cereals. Our skin makes vitamin D when it reacts to sunlight hitting its surface. Sunscreen is recommended to prevent skin cancers, however, in order to get adequate vitamin D, it is recommended that you spend 20 minutes a day outside on bright days without sunscreen, at least twice a week. If you live someplace that has bouts of limited sunshine, it is recommended that you not wear sunglasses on cloudy days in order to absorb as much sun as possible, because chances are on those days it is also cold and the rest of your body is all bundled up.

The current RDA for vitamin D is 400 IU, however, most research is revealing that this level is not sufficient. Most studies do not show beneficial effects of vitamin D in disease prevention until the levels reached are in the region of 1,000 to 2,000 IU. In the near future, the RDA level for this vitamin may be expanded. Vitamin D3 is the most easily and readily assimilated form of vitamin D supplement.

Vitamin E

Another super antioxidant, vitamin E is necessary for many bodily functions, such as tissue repair and growth, blood healing, maintenance of healthy nerves and muscles, the promotion of healthy hair, skin and nails, relaxation of leg cramps, and the reduction of scar tissue, among other things. It aids in the prevention of numerous conditions, including cellular damage, cancer (including prostate and breast), cardiovascular disease, and high blood pressure. In all, vitamin E has been shown to protect against more than 80 diseases and medical conditions.

Dietary sources are brown rice, cold pressed vegetable oils, dark green and leafy vegetables, eggs, peas and legumes, milk, nuts, seeds (including flax), and other whole grains, like corn meal.

That's it for the vitamin portion. We only go through the first part of the alphabet, and for more information it is well worth it to invest in a Nutritional Almanac. *Staying Healthy with Nutrition, 21st Century Edition*, is a very good one and was co-written by one of my beloved instructors from Bastyr University, Buck Levin.

Water and salt

Most of the material absorbed from the cavity of the small intestine is water in which salt is dissolved. The salt and water come from the food and liquid we swallow and the juices secreted by the many digestive glands. Yes, we do need some salt in our diets, but not nearly as much as our tastes buds have acquired a liking for.

- **Water** – Our bodies are made up of about 60 to 70 percent water. It is just as vital to our health as the air we breathe, which is why some experts will say that water is the most the important nutrient you consume. It is involved in almost every function of the body. Water is responsible for transporting all the nutrients, oxygen and waste products in and out of cells. It lubricates organs, tissues and joints, and helps to regulate our body temperature.

  o We all know we need to drink water every day, but how much? One method to determine how much water you need is by dividing your body weight (in kg) by 30. So for example, if you weigh 120 lbs (divided by 2.2 = ~ 55 kg), 55 x 30 = 1650 ml, that means you should drink about 55 ounces (multiply ml by .034 to get ounces), or about 7 cups (there are 8 ounces in a cup) of water a day.

  o This doesn't mean to rush out and drink all that water at once. In fact, it is recommended that you drink the water 2 or 3 ounces at a time and in-between meals. If you drink too much with a meal, it can dilute your digestive enzymes. It doesn't really matter if it's warm or ice cold, drink it however you like, just drink it. Some frames work better with warm water, for instance, Skys should drink their water warm.

- **Salt** – Our bodies have a physiological requirement for sodium, and salt (sodium chloride) is our main dietary source of sodium. Yes, our bodies need it, but on average, our intake is significantly higher than our need. Most people are able to deal with the excess by excreting it, but some people are sensitive to it and prone to high blood pressure. The elderly are more sensitive to excess sodium and therefore at greater risk for high blood pressure.

o In the U.S. we do not have a daily recommended value for sodium. Many experts suggest salt intake should not exceed 5 grams (or 5,000 mg) a day (or 2 grams of sodium). However, that still seems high, so if you can try to keep your intake to no more than 2,400 mg, which is about one (1) teaspoon of table salt. This includes all sodium from foods and what's added while cooking. Some think it should be lower, and in the UK, the daily value is 1,600 mg.

Phytonutrients:

Think of these as ground troops, they fight (phyte) disease by blocking free radical damage to our cells. Free radicals are very reactive, unstable molecules that hang around our cells for a short period of time. But, in that time, they can do a lot of damage if they react with other molecules. When free radicals interact with various compounds in a cell, the combination can initiate cancer, DNA mutations, atherosclerosis, as well as autoimmune and coronary heart diseases. Phytonutrients can be found in fruits and vegetables. Each fruit and vegetable has its own distinct color and each color represents a different phytonutrient. For example, the blue in blueberries gives them the power to do many amazing things for our bodies, including helping to boost collagen, which keeps our skin cells strong.

Antioxidants

(Free) Radical damage is a given because they are the result of normal metabolic processes and our body's reaction to infection. Therefore, little can be done to prevent their formation. However, since the main tissue damaging radicals are called oxygen radicals, the compounds that protect against oxygen radicals are called antioxidants. The main antioxidants that come from our food supply are:

Vitamin E – high doses of vitamin E may protect against atherosclerosis and heart disease.
Carotenes (Beta Carotene and Vitamin A) – high blood levels of carotene have been shown to be associated with low incidence of a variety of cancers.
Vitamin C – vitamin C can act on the surface of cells to prevent damage, which is why it is said to affect the results of aging, i.e. prevent or minimize wrinkles.

*** *Many clinical trials show that high blood levels of these vitamins from supplements may have actually caused types of cancers and increased mortality, so overdoing supplementation is never recommended. Tell your doctor if you take any supplements.*

Fruits and Vegetables

Fruits and vegetables have a combination of the above antioxidants, macro, micro, and phyto- nutrients. They should cover most of your lunch and dinner plates. They have all the nutrients we need and should be the basis of our diets. With the economy the way it is, think about growing your own vegetables. It's a great activity for kids, too: they love it! You don't even need a lot of space; you can have a kitchen garden using buckets, and this is a great way to grow herbs. Lettuce is also very easy, quick and fun to grow!

I received the chart below in an email and added to it. It makes a very compelling argument as to why we should ingest more of nature's wonderful gifts. Maybe we should look for more clues from nature on how to feed and heal our bodies...

Mother Nature has given us many clues as to which foods help what part of our bodies:

A sliced <u>Carrot</u> looks like the human eye. The pupil, iris and radiating lines look just like the human eye... and YES, science now shows carrots greatly enhance blood flow to and function of the eyes.

A <u>Tomato</u> has four chambers and is red. The heart has four chambers and is red. Research shows tomatoes are loaded with lycopine and are indeed pure heart and blood food.

Grapes hang in a cluster that has the shape of the heart. Each grape looks like a blood cell and research today shows grapes are also profound heart and blood vitalizing food.

A Walnut looks like a little brain, a left and right hemisphere, upper cerebrums and lower cerebellums. Even the wrinkles or folds on the nut are just like the neo-cortex. We now know walnuts help develop more than three (3) dozen neuron-transmitters for brain function.

Kidney Beans actually heal and help maintain kidney function and yes, they look exactly like the human kidneys.

Celery, Bok Choy, Rhubarb and many more look just like bones. These foods specifically target bone strength. Bones are 23% sodium and these foods are 23% sodium. If you don't have enough sodium in your diet, the body pulls it from the bones, thus making them weak. These foods replenish the skeletal needs of the body.

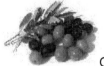 Avocadoes, Eggplants, and Pears target the health and function of the womb and cervix of the female – and they look just like these organs. Today's research shows that when a woman eats one avocado a week, it balances hormones, sheds unwanted birth weight, and prevents cervical cancer. And how profound is this? It takes exactly nine (9) months to grow an avocado from blossom to ripened fruit. There are more than 14,000 photolytic chemical constituents of nutrition in each one of these foods (modern science has only studied and named about 141 of them).

Figs are full of seeds and hang in twos when they grow. Figs increase the mobility of male sperm and increase the numbers of sperm as well to overcome male sterility. They resemble the male testicles.

Sweet Potatoes look like the pancreas and actually balance the glycemic index of diabetics.

Olives assist the health and function of the ovaries.

Oranges, Grapefruits, and other Citrus fruits look just like the mammary glands of the female and actually assist the health of the breasts and the movement of lymph in and out of the breasts.

Onions look like the body's cells. Today's research shows onions help clear waste materials from all of the body cells. They even produce tears which wash the epithelial layers of the eyes. A working companion, Garlic, also helps eliminate waste materials and dangerous free radicals from the body.

Pomegranate looks like a female breast and it is very good for firming breast tissue and may help reduce the risk of breast cancer.

Nature is our best pharmacy!

Whole Foods

What are whole foods, anyway? Shouldn't all foods be whole? What's the other stuff if only whole foods are whole? Half? Part? Hmmm, maybe...

Whole foods are foods found in their most natural whole state. Until the last century, and mostly the last 50 or so years, humans survived predominately on whole foods found in nature. In fact, a recent study explains that over the last 10,000 years humans ate virtually the same thing and that it has only been during the last 50 decades (500 years) that our diets wavered from that. With the rise of industrialization and agribusiness came the attraction and popularity of refined, processed foods.

With all of these refined foods, there have been a slew of health problems, like obesity, heart disease, high cholesterol, and high blood pressure. Thankfully, we are beginning to realize that eating whole foods is the way our bodies were meant to eat. Deep down, we know that whole, fresh, and natural foods are the best nourishment for our bodies. Think about the children. Shouldn't that be especially so for little growing bodies?

Look at the current state of the health of our children and you'll see that changing the way we eat is critical. Children born today are the first generation in America to have a shorter life expectancy than their parents! 45% of children are at increased risk for obesity related diseases, 30 % of children ages 6 to 19 are overweight and 15% are obese. With obesity comes the higher prevalence of diabetes, hypertension, and orthopedic complications for these youngsters.

We all have our own ideas of what whole foods, or wholesomeness is and what it isn't and I think it's fair to say that a highly processed, pre-packaged "snack" lunch is not exactly wholesome.

When I picture my body, my vehicle I think of what it would have been like 1,000 years ago before fast food and microwaves. I imagine the kinds of foods available would be things I either gathered from my surroundings, or hunted for. I probably would have found lots of fresh green things and other colorful sweet, crunchy things to eat too. The human body hasn't changed in it's most basic nutritional needs, the human diet has changed dramatically in the last 100 to even 50 years.

A well-balanced diet: *Okay, so what is a well-balanced diet?*   On average, women need about 2,000 calories and men need 2,500 calories per day. These calories need to come from the macronutrients we discussed earlier, from healthy, hearty, natural foods that that were designed to run the human frame. The reason our bodies have gotten so out of balance is that each day America's over-productive food supply produces 3,900 calories per person. There is a huge gap between what we need and what's available to us. Because of this abundance, the food producers must think up ways to get us to purchase and consume all these extra calories. Many of the items on the grocery shelf and in fast food joints are highly refined and are there solely because they yield a high profit margin, not because of their health benefits. The biggest culprit is high-fructose corn syrup (America consumes a staggering 83 pounds per person each year!). Next up is aspartame, Splenda, pesticides, hormones, antibiotics, preservatives, dyes, fillers, stabilizers and other chemical creations. Because our bodies, our machines do not know what to do with these items, our body either needs to eliminate them or store them. This dilemma is what's steering our body vehicles onto the fast lane to the highway to the hospital. We need to hop on the highway to health!

No matter how you slice it, ounce-for-ounce and calorie-for-calorie, nutrient-dense, fiber-rich whole foods are more filling and more nutritious! Many of the highly refined foods contain empty calories. Empty calories fill you up very well, but they provide no nutritional value. If you take something wholesome, fresh and real like an apple, a baked potato, or a grilled salmon filet, every calorie is productively used by the body's engine.

The following diagram shows what kinds of foods make up a wholesome diet. At the base of wheel is Fresh, Local, Seasonal, and Organic, foods in this state are most likely to be the ones that your body, your vehicle were developed to consume and are what make it run smoothly, with less dinging and knocking. In her book, *Feeding the Whole Family*, Cynthia Liar has a really nice hand written diagram.

A well-balanced diet contains:

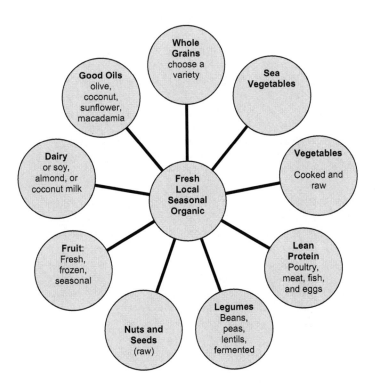

Staples – A well-balanced kitchen starts with:

- Main dishes: Grains, beans, vegetables, and fruit are the key to a whole foods diet and are absolutely critical to a vegetarian or vegan diet. Humans have eaten these foods for millennium and it is time to return to them as a staple in the modern diet. They are packed with nutrients and rich in fiber.
- Whole grains: The whole grains contain protein, fiber (the bran part of the plant), B vitamins, calcium, iron, vitamin E and the germ (which is the reproductive, or life giving part of the plant). Refined varieties (white bread, rice and pasta) have none of this, just sprayed on vitamins which are usually cooked or rinsed off.

- o Amaranth
- o Brown Rice
- o Buckwheat (toasted = kasha)
- o Hulled barley
- o Millet
- o Oats
- o Quinoa
- o Spelt
- o Sweet brown rice

If you've never heard of some of these grains, try them! You can usually purchase them at any store that sells bulk grains. Remember to rotate grains in your diet, as eating too much of one grain for too long a period can create a sensitivity to it. Hence, the increased wheat intolerances we are experiencing in this country.

- Legumes: beans, peas, lentils, and soy products. Beans are rich in complex carbs and protein, high in fiber and low in calories. For centuries, many cultures have paired whole grains with legumes, because they complement each other's proteins; most grains lack one amino acid (lysine), while most beans lack another (methionine). Together they make a complete protein. Vegetarians usually pay attention to this and try to combine their proteins. They do not, however, have to be combined in the same meal, but it's best if they are eaten in the same day.
  - o Black beans
  - o Brown lentils
  - o Cannellini beans
  - o Christmas lima beans
  - o French lentils
  - o Chickpeas (garbanzos)
  - o Kidney beans
  - o Navy beans
  - o Pinto beans
  - o Red lentils
  - o Split peas

- Soy Products: Soy has gotten a lot of attention for its health benefits and many companies have started making soy everything, even soy candy bars (a.k.a "energy bars"). The news is getting grimmer about the truth behind soy's magic. I have read some credible scientific studies that tell tales of adverse effects from eating too many processed soy products (such as fake meats and cheeses, protein drinks, etc...) including breast cancer, early puberty, retarded growth in children, sexual dysfunction, and thyroid deficiencies: the list goes on. We don't know for sure what the effect of all these highly processed items could be, but I say we should play it safe. We do know that soy has more phytic acid than other beans, which can affect mineral and protein absorption.

- o   When considering eating soy products, we should take heed from the culture that probably uses the most soy products: Japan. Throughout many centuries of trial and error, they have found ways to healthfully use soybeans: They ferment it, as in tamari (soy sauce), shoyu (another sauce), miso and tempeh. Ironically or not, cultures that traditionally use soy products in their diets also use sea vegetables. This is a way to combine nutrients similar to protein combining; sea vegetables would counter any effects of mineral absorption and thyroid problems due to the soy because of the abundance of minerals and iodine in the sea veggies.
  - ▪   We noted in Chapter One that there has been a rise in hypo thyroid cases, soy products are hard on the thyroid, sea vegetables ease the thyroid so the pair together well.
- o   Soy has phytoestrogens and is recommended for peri, pre and post menopausal women. These phytoestrogens help ease women in mid life with her discomfort, however they may be harmful to a young girl's or boy's growing body.
- o   If you choose to eat soy products, remember the whole foods creed, the less processed, the more whole the food is.

These are the safest soy products to consume:
- ▪   Miso
- ▪   Shoyu
- ▪   Tamari
- ▪   Tempeh
- ▪   Tofu (tofu is not a fermented soy product, although it is often served with fermented soy products. The phytic acid of the soybean, which is hard on the human system, is mostly found in the fiber, and is excluded from the tofu making process).

Buy dry beans and grains in bulk; it saves on packaging and cost. You can store them in a dark place and in clear glass jars (that's what you can do with those empty spaghetti sauce jars).

- Vegetables: We should eat both cooked and raw vegetables daily, this helps mix things up a bit. Cooking lessens some of the nutritional value, but makes it easier to digest. Raw veggies are rich in nutrients and some enzymes are lost in cooking (broccoli and cauliflower are harder to digest raw). The USDA has a motto that I love "Eat the Rainbow." Eat all the colors every day or at least every week. Dark green and orange veggies should be eaten every day!
  - Arugula
  - Beets/ beet greens
  - Bok Choy
  - Broccoli
  - Cabbage
  - Carrots
  - Chard
  - Chinese cabbage
  - Collards
  - Kale
  - Leaf lettuce
  - Mustard greens
  - Potatoes
  - Spinach
  - Sweet potatoes
  - Swiss chard
  - Watercress
  - Winter squash
  - Yams

- Fruit: Choosing in-season fruit is the most cost effective and delicious. Consider stocking up and freezing it. Cooked and dried fruits are good choices and frozen fruit is great, too. Dry fruits are especially good in winter time and are my favorite. I eat dried fruits to curb my sweet tooth and, paired with nuts and seeds, they make great alternatives to "energy bars."

  - Apples
  - Apricots
  - Blueberries
  - Cranberries

- o   Dates
- o   Grapes
- o   Kiwis
- o   Lemons
- o   Melons
- o   Oranges
- o   Papaya
- o   Pears
- o   Persimmons
- o   Pomegranate
- o   Plums
- o   Raisins
- o   Raspberries
- o   Strawberries
- o   Tomatoes

Food Allergies and Intolerances

I could write an entire book on food allergies and intolerances, but there are plenty of good books already out there about that subject, so I'm not going to get into too much detail here. I do want to touch on this subject, because it seems that food intolerances are on the rise and more and more people are avoiding products like wheat, eggs, dairy, nuts and soy. Your body makes antibodies to kill harmful substances. When you have an intolerance or allergy, sometimes your body attacks harmless ones like food. It's difficult to determine if you're having a reaction to food, because so often the symptoms are subtle and creep up over years and years of time.

We can even crave and become addicted to the food to which we've become intolerant.   When we eat the food to which we have an intolerance, we may feel a lift after eating it because the body is producing adrenaline to fight the reaction. After a couple of hours, the feeling goes away and eventually the body wears down from all the stimulation and we need more of the food to feel good again. This can be like any addiction. The most common substance we associate this to is caffeine. Many people can't live without their morning cup of coffee, but what they don't realize is that it may not be just the addictive qualities of the caffeine itself they're craving, caffeine can be an allergenic.

There are many reasons we have allergies and intolerances and the reasons are not completely understood. One thing for sure is that they are on the rise. This is probably due to all the pollutants, chemically treated food and water, and prescription medicines we're taking into our bodies. Our skin is also exposed to many toxic substances. The food we eat is produced with pesticides, mycotoxins, dyes, additives, preservatives, fillers, binders and uber-sugars. We have heavy metals in our teeth and in the fumes we inhale every day. Our livers and defense systems have become stressed and over-worked and are failing to be efficient.

The way our food is produced today, in factory farms that use chemical fertilizers and pesticides, mass production, long distance transportation, long-term storage, and convenience cooking can lead to a decrease in valuable nutrients within the food supply and ultimately nutritional deficiencies. These vitamins and minerals are necessary for proper immune function. A poor immune system can lead to allergies, so it is a vicious cycle.

If you eat a lot of refined sugar, wheat and milk products (like so many of us), you may be a target for food intolerances, because the aforementioned deplete vitamins and minerals from your body. For example, the raw molasses extracted from sugar cane actually has vitamins and minerals that our bodies need to digest the sugars. Unfortunately, most of us eat refined white sugar, which doesn't have any of the nutrients we need to metabolize it, so the body draws on its reserves. Wheat and sugar can also promote the growth of too many unfriendly bacteria called *Candida albicans*. Candida is yeast that lives inside and outside the body. Normally it stays in check by the "friendly flora" in the intestines. However, when the immune system is suppressed, Candida can grow out of control and damage the intestinal lining, allowing food particles to pass through the intestinal walls, triggering intolerances. Similarly, wheat (gluten) and milk can also coat the intestinal lining and damage it in much the same way. Because we're eating milk, sugar and wheat at nearly every meal (this wasn't the case 50 year ago), it's no wonder intolerances to these items are on the rise.

What foods cause reactions? The foods listed below are most likely to be causing you, or a loved one, problems. Beware: sometimes it's tough to tell in children, severe eczema (blotchy, itchy, red skin), stomach pain, and mood swings could be a sign of food intolerance; consult a healthcare professional if you detect a problem. Because many grains and items we normally eat can cause sensitivities, many doctors, nutritionists, and naturopaths recommend more variety in the diet. It is suggested that we not eat wheat every day, three times a day. We should mix other grains in, as well, so that we don't overload our systems. It's worth a try, especially if you detect a possible sensitivity. The best way to know for sure is to eliminate that item from your diet for a while and bring it back in. There is a science to that method, so seek assistance if you're going to start an elimination diet.

The foods that cause most allergies/ intolerances:

Apples
Cane and beet sugar
Citrus fruits
Coffee (caffeine)
Corn
Soy
Dairy products
Eggs
Food additives and preservatives (try to avoid highly processed foods)
Garlic
Gluten (wheat, barley, rye, oats [oats don't have gluten but are often processed on the same machinery so pick up the residue])
Leeks
Onions
Peanuts
Shellfish
Strawberries
Tap water
Tea (black/ caffeinated)
Tomatoes & Potatoes (and other members of the Nightshade family such as sweet and hot peppers, eggplant, tomatillos, tamarios, pepinos, pimentos, paprika, cayenne, and hot sauces. Nightshades have alkaloids which many people react to)

Know Your Taste Buds

Your tongue is an organ and a major facilitator for digestion. Did you know there are 16 muscles in the tongue? Our tongues do a lot for us, we can lick with it, touch with it, and taste with it. It is filled with nerves which gives us many pleasurable sensations. There are actually thousands of taste buds on the tongue where the tastes are picked up. We only identify Six Tastes and each has a special spot on our tongues where they flourish, we call them **Taste Buds**. Each taste bud has receptor cells that send messages to the brain through sensory nerves.

Your taste buds require certain tastes to alert your stomach and the rest of your digestive tract to what's coming. If you are American, the chances are your taste buds would like you to liven them up, a lot! Do them a favor and invite them to sample more of the foods they were designed to enjoy. With such a range available to us, it is a pity so many of us don't enjoy more tastes and variety in our diet. Our bodies would actually thank us for it if we did and we would feel much better for it!

Our tongues have Six Tastes, in six locations: Sweet, Salty, Sour, Bitter, Pungent and Astringent. Our digestive process as a whole requires these six tastes to function properly. Most traditional cultural foods around the world incorporate these six tastes to awaken the senses and get the bodies' "juices flowing."

Knowing your taste buds and building your diet based on your palate is like choosing the right octane fuel for your car's engine. Think of your body like a high performance engine, and just like a car, it runs better with less knocking, on high octane fuel. High octane fuel for your body is full of flavor and color. Experiment with the different herbs and spices that give our food such wonderful flavors and textures.

In order to enliven your taste buds, get to know your tongue a little better. Take a look at it in the mirror, what does it say about you and your diet? Practitioners of Traditional Chinese Medicine (TCM) and Ayurveda can tell a lot about you and your diet by looking at your tongue!

Let's look at two different pictures of the tongue and their taste buds: (my apologies, these pictures are not very clear)

Western:

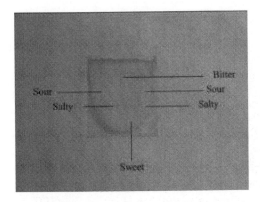

Eastern:

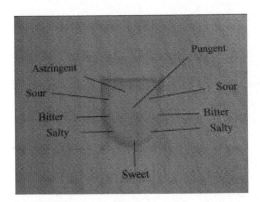

They are similar, aren't they? The main difference is that the Western diagram doesn't include **Pungent** or **Astringent** on the tongue. *Why do you think that is?* Cleary we can taste spicy, pungent foods like hot chili peppers. We can also taste astringent flavors in potatoes and beans.

> *"Kisa Gotami lost her mind when her child died. The disconsolate mother begged of the Buddha to awaken the baby. The compassionate Buddha asked her to fetch some mustard from any house where death had not taken place. With high hopes she visited street after street and when she could not find a single house where death had not taken place, she understood the universality of death. She became a nun and a saint."*

The Buddha did not tell Kisa to seek American hotdog mustard, or Dijon for that matter. What she searched for was a spice, most likely in the form of a seed or ground into a yellowy powder. This powerful story comes from India where there are many different herbs and spices used for cooking. Scientists are discovering that many of the herbs and spices used in Indian cuisine have profound medicinal properties. For instance, University of Arizona scientists have found that turmeric, a spice in many Indian dishes helps ease inflammation and may fight arthritis.

Color Your Palate

Now that you're more familiar with your tongue and its taste buds, it's time to tickle them! Eat all the colors of the rainbow in order to color your palate and refuel your system.

Fruits and vegetables come in all those beautiful colors and each color has its own special nutrients that are so good for us. Eating the colors of the rainbow helps you stay healthy and is really fun. You can make shish-kabobs with veggies and pineapple and grill or bake them, you can mix veggies, quinoa and dried fruits up in a salad, and you can shake up fruit into a smoothie!

Each color of vegetable has its own phytonutrient which gives us power and energy and helps us fight (phyt) disease. We are so lucky, too, because they taste great, especially when you prepare them with all the tantalizing herbs and spices we have!

It's fun and easy to make good healthy food using lots of vibrant, organic vegetables. To help you start incorporating more of the six tastes into your diet and color your palate everyday, use the herbs and spices on your Frames list.

> **A great way to try new foods and get new ideas is to choose what foods you want to prepare, or some random items you have on hand and Google them to see what interesting recipes pop up. Try it, you'll like it!**

Digestion and the Six Tastes

As we've learned, digestion is very important, therefore, the foods we consume are very important. Each of the six tastes has a part of digestion that it represents and foods that affect it. Some foods are better for certain frames than others, which means they keep the frame balanced: think of it as wheel alignment. If you hit a curb, your steering could be off, and while it won't keep your car from running, it won't run as smoothly.

Same with foods, if you eat foods that knock your frame out of balance, your body won't run as smoothly. Your frame could be so far out of balance that you don't even notice, until you get a tune-up and feel the difference. Try sticking to foods that balance your frame and limiting the ones that don't.

The Six Tastes and their roles in digestion:

1. Sweet - Starts in the mouth.
- Sweet foods nourish, cool, moisten, oil, and increase weight.
  - Milk, rice, wheat, sugar, syrup, honey, dates, licorice (root), sweet or dried fruits and vegetables, starches, fats, oils, carbs
    - **These foods increase Moon**
    - **They decrease Sky and Sun**

2. Sour – Stomach area, where enzymes are secreted and fat and protein start getting broken down.
- Sour foods warm, oil, and increase weight
  - Citrus fruits, yogurt, pickles, some cheeses, sour cream, green grapes, strawberry, alcohol, fermented food, soy sauce, miso.
    - **Theses foods increase Sun and Moon**
    - **They decrease Sky**

3. Salty – Duodenum (a place where the stomach attaches to the jejunum (upper small intestine). Bile salts secreted, carbohydrate, protein, and fat digested, electrolytes balance.
- Salty foods warm, dissolve, stimulate, soften, oil, and increase weight

- Salt (sea salt, rock salt, mineral salts), cucumber, zucchini, tomatoes, celery, electrolytes.
  - **These foods increase Sun and Moon**
  - **They decrease Sky**

4. Bitter - Jejunum (small intestine) more enzymes released, enhanced circulation.
  - Bitter foods cool, dry, purify and decrease weight
    - Coffee, black tea, Aloe Vera, lettuce, endive, dandelion, turmeric, rhubarb
      - **These foods increase Sky**
      - **They decrease Sun and Moon**

5. Pungent - Ileum (lower small intestine), rapid absorption, cools body, lightens stomach.
  - Pungent foods warm, dry, stimulate, and decrease weight
    - Cayenne, chili, black pepper, onion, garlic, mustard, radish, basil, oregano, sage, ginger, basil, bay leaves.
      - **These foods increase Sun**
      - **They decrease Sky and Moon**

6. Astringent - Waste enters rectum, feces formed and eliminated, hunger returns.
  - Astringent foods cool, dry, reduce stickiness
    - Green apples, unripe banana, pomegranate, okra, potatoes, chickpeas, beans, lentils, green beans, sprouts, turmeric, which hazel.
      - **These foods increase Sky and Moon**
      - **They decrease Sun**

Everyone needs some of each of the six tastes. The more of the tastes you include in a meal, the better it is for you. By incorporating all the tastes in every meal, it kick-starts the enzymes needed for digestion and gets the whole process started.

Taste starts your system and lets your body know what's coming. It's like turning your key in the ignition. You have to start the engine before you can get moving.

Look at some common foods around the globe and what tastes they include:

Western
- **French** – Baguette and Brie, Wine = Sweet, Sour, Astringent
- **Spanish Speaking–** Beans, Rice and Tortillas = Astringent, Sweet, Pungent
- **American** – Apple Pie or Burger and Fries (Hot Dog? Corn Dog?) = Sweet and Salty

Eastern
- **Japanese** – Sushi, Soy Sauce, and Seaweed = Astringent, Sweet, Salty, Bitter
- **Indian** – Curry and Saffron Rice = Sweet, Salty, Sour, Bitter, Astringent, Pungent
- **Chinese** – Stir-Fry and Tofu = Astringent, Sweet, Salty, Pungent

---

Food and Culture

We need food to function, which is why food is so important to everyone. Some people say that food defines a culture; each culture definitely has its own delicacies and customs. Within almost every society, people have developed ways to approach food and how it is converted into energy in the body. Ironically, most of them are remarkably similar, yet they do have differences.

Let's look at some of the similarities and differences regarding food and digestion between some of the countries within the two major medical philosophies:

What do these food/mealtime sayings say about their culture?

Western
- **French** –*Bon Appetit* = *Good Appetite*
- **Spanish** - *Buen Provecho* = *Good Digestion*
- **American** – *"Down the hatch"* or *"Dig in"*

Eastern
- **Japanese** – *"Itadakimasu"* = *Humbly receive*
- **Indian** – *"Ann Brahma"* = Sanskrit for food, means *"God"*
- **Chinese** – *"Dim sum"* = A common snack, means *"Touch the heart"*

Some dishes to try and their country of origin:

- Tiebou dienne – Senegal
- Peanut stew– Ghana
- Pad Thai – Thailand
- Dahl – India
- Pho - Vietnam
- Hummus – Middle East
- Dolmas - Mediterranean
- Herbal Tea - try a variety of warm herbal teas to drink. Many of the herbs have healing properties, antioxidants, and astringent or bitter tastes that are good for our tongues and digestion.

Do the above traditional foods satisfy the needs of the three body frames?

It's time to mix things up and enjoy new tastes, try different herbs and spices! Some you'll like and some you won't, but it'll be a good experience either way! Learn a little about the culture from which the blend of spices comes.

Here is my recipe for herbal chai tea of Indian origin; it is balancing for all frame types and delicious: Experiment with your own amounts, some may like more ginger, some more cinnamon, etc...

My Chai Tea*

Ingredients:
2 -3 slices fresh ginger
5 whole cloves
7 cardamom pods
1 stick of cinnamon
2 star anise
Pinch (about 5) fenugreek seeds
5 black pepper corns (those needing to decrease Sun may not want to include the peppercorn)

* *adjust the amount of each spice to your liking*

Method:
Boil a pot of water (about 4 cups), put all the ingredients into the boiling water, cover and remove from heat, steep for about 5 to 10 minutes. Ladle into cups or strain liquid into a tea pot. Can be served as is or with milk (dairy, rice, almond, coconut, or soy) and a touch of honey.

When purchasing spices, try to buy them in bulk, many groceries stores and most health food stores have a section for bulk spices. You can save several dollars per spice by buying them this way – usually what you're paying for is the container. If you have old spice jars that are empty, reuse them. I buy my spices in bulk, make my own labels and store them in clean, dry baby food jars, so my cinnamon costs me a few pennies verses $4.00!

> **Children love tea and it's good for them! It provides healthy antioxidants unlike a soda pop. As long as it is lukewarm and caffeine free (like the one above) children can drink it. Theirs should be more dilute (with water or a small amount of juice) than an adult portion.**

Think about your diet, what are the tastes you eat most?

As a professional, I have seen that Americans eat mostly Sweet, Salty and the occasional Sour and Pungent foods. These usually come in extreme doses. I attribute much of our food choices to the food supply in

America, over-production of certain foods based on ease for mass consumption and maximum profit. There is an over abundance of overweight in our society, and, as a culture, our collective Moon is out of balance. If you look at many traditional, native cultures, overweight and obesity is almost non-existent.   Yet in America over 50% of our population is currently overweight.

Unfortunately, the lack of variety in the American diet has been proving to be the root of a major health crisis. Perhaps this is something we should take more seriously, especially when you consider the roles the Six Tastes play in digestion and the overall health of our bodies as a system.

When it comes to your body as your vehicle, you only get one in this world; you can't trade it in for another one. So, you might as well give it what it requires to run efficiently. I think you'll find that it feels great to nourish your body the way it is meant to be nourished and you'll most likely stay a lot healthier, too.

If you try something new and it is a strange, unfamiliar taste, don't give up, research shows it takes 4 days for your tongue to develop a 'taste' for something new or different. Don't give up, try the herb or spice again the next day, in a new way.

Children often have a hard time trying new things, research shows that young palates can require seven to twelve exposures to a new taste before they get used to it and begin to enjoy it. Keep trying!

Portion Distortion

A little bit of a good thing is still a good thing! We don't have to get all crazy and eat more than one human portion.   What is one human portion? Well, if you keep in mind that your stomach is about the size of your fist then you'll see that we really aren't meant to eat a whole lot more than that in one sitting. Overeating is not much different than over drinking, it is still an addiction. Once you cross that point and eat more than one brownie and you go back for three or four brownies, it's too much, and is more than one human portion.

It's time to be mindful of our portions and what we're eating. In Sanskrit, food means God and that gives me something to think about. We should treat our food with respect and be mindful about what kinds of food we're choosing, how we prepare it, how we eat it and how much of it we eat. Think of food as a type of **meditation** or prayer to our bodies. Make it peaceful and beautiful, something of which to be proud and to worship.

Portion sizes

If you look at portion sizes from 20 years ago versus today, you'll see what a huge (pun intended) difference there is in the portions of food being served and eaten. The size of a hamburger, piece of pizza, tub of popcorn, and soda have all doubled - or more!

I love to tell this story to my classes and clients... When my mom was a little girl (she was born in 1939), every couple of months, she and her two brothers would get enough money from their aunt to buy a soda pop. They would go to the diner and buy one 10 ounce bottle of orange drink and share it. She remembers how they would line up the three clear glasses on the counter and pour out the drink to make sure it was evenly distributed among the siblings. Think about that in today's standards when many kids have several 12 ounce cans of soda all to themselves, every day. Times have certainly changed and not always for the better.

Here are some items around the house that you can compare to know what one human portion really ought to be:

Item	Should be this size
Bagel	Can of tuna
Brownie	Dental floss package
Butter	1 poker chip
Cereal	Baseball
Cheese	6 dice
Cookie	2 poker chips
Grilled fish	Checkbook
Mashed potatoes	Light bulb
Meat	Deck of cards (or palm of your hand)
Nuts	Golf ball
Pancake or tortilla	CD/DVD
Peanut butter	Thumb nail (no larger than golf ball)
Potato	Computer mouse
Raw vegetables	Fist
¼ cup dried fruit or nuts	Golf ball or large egg
1 cup ice cream	Tennis ball

Food Additives and Preservatives
They're everywhere, but what are they, anyway?

Additive

Basically, a food additive is any substance that is *added* to food. The legal definition from the Food and Drug Administration (FDA) is "any substance the intended use which results or may reasonably be expected to result-directly or indirectly-in its becoming a component or otherwise affecting the characteristics of any food." This also includes any substance used in the production, processing, treatment, packaging, transportation or storage of food.

Natural and chemical substances are added to foods for many reasons:
- ✓ to give it a longer shelf
- ✓ so it taste better
- ✓ to give it better mouth feel (palatability)

> **It's no coincidence that two of the three main reasons for additives have to do with our tongue!**

There are more than 3,000 additives approved by the Food and Drug Administration. An additive may be deemed safe, but manufacturers don't always have to list all additives on food labels.

In 1958, the FDA approved The Food Additives Amendment to the FD&C Act; it requires FDA approval before an additive can be included in food. There are a couple of loopholes in this amendment:

- It leaves the responsibility to prove an additive's safety up to the manufacturer. If the governing party is not overseeing safety testing, and leaving it up to the producer to judge safety, it's easy to see where problems can arise.
- The Food Additives Amendment exempted two groups of substances from the food additive regulation process:
  1. All substances that FDA or USDA had determined were safe for use in specific foods prior to the 1958 amendment were designated as "prior-sanctioned substances." Some examples of prior-sanctioned substances are sodium nitrite and potassium nitrite used to preserve hot dogs, cold cuts, etc. In 2010, these

products have numerous research findings to suggest they are linked to many forms of cancer.

2. Products deemed generally recognized as safe or GRAS substances are also excluded. GRAS substances are generally recognized as safe by experts, based on their history of use in food before 1958 or based on published scientific evidence. Salt, sugar, spices, vitamins and monosodium glutamate are on the GRAS list, as well as several hundred other substances. Manufacturers can request the FDA to review a substance to determine if it is GRAS.

> **Food coloring is an additive**

There has been a lot of public concern regarding the safety of food additives, namely food colorings, therefore, the U.S. Department of Agriculture (USDA) made the Food Additives and Color Additives Amendment. It prohibits the approval of an additive if it is found to cause cancer in humans or animals. This clause is commonly referred to as the Delaney Clause, named for its Congressional sponsor, Rep. James Delaney (D-N.Y.). At the time, there were 200 color additives listed as GRAS, 90 of them remain on the GRAS list, the remainder have been removed from use by the FDA or have been withdrawn by industry.

Even with the rigors of testing and regulation, many of the color additives that continue to be used in food are controversial and continue to pose health risks. The USDA's response is that because artificial color additives used in food are mandated to be listed on product labels, like FD&C yellow #5, people who wish to avoid consuming them may do so. So, read thy label! Please note: natural coloring additives do not have to be listed as an ingredient, so coloring agents like crushed beetles may not be on your ingredient list! We'll discuss more about label reading in the next chapter.

> **Enriched**

The processing of wheat and grain products causes many of their natural nutrients to be lost. Therefore, manufacturers replace the lost nutrients by adding chemical ingredients in an attempt to *enrich* them with the lost vitamins and minerals. For instance, when rice is hulled and all the bran removed, many of the crucial B vitamins are also removed. Food manufacturers literally spray chemical vitamins back onto the rice and thus it is "enriched" with an additive. The sad part is, because the natural vitamin is no longer a part of the rice, much of the added vitamin is washed off during cooking and not ingested. That is why rinsing enriched grain products (most white rice and pasta) is not recommended. If you rinse them off, you won't get some of the vitamins that are disclosed on the nutrition facts panel.

Any time you buy a box of enriched product, you are buying a product whose natural source of nutrients was destroyed in processing; a chemical was added to it to replace the nutritional value.

> ➤ **Fortified**

Fortification is the process by which a manufacturer adds a chemical or substance to increase its nutritional content with a nutrient that may not have been naturally occurring. For instance, iodine is added to salt to prevent goiter in the United States. Many breakfast cereals are fortified with added vitamins and minerals to boost their nutritional content.

Preservatives

Preservatives do just what the name implies, they preserve food. They keep bacteria and molds from growing on breads and meats and prevent oils (like salad dressings) from becoming rancid for a very long time. Essentially, they prolong the shelf life of products, so that a box of biscuit mix can stay on the shelf for years and not be rancid. Preservatives are not there to make you healthier.

Preservatives must be listed on ingredient labels by their common or usual names on all foods that contain them -- which are most processed food.

The USDA states on the worldwide web that; *"Unless you grow all your food in your own garden and prepare all your meals from scratch, it's almost impossible to eat food without preservatives added by manufacturers during processing... You'll see calcium propionate on most bread labels, disodium EDTA on canned kidney beans, and BHA on shortening, just to name a few. Even snack foods--dried fruit, potato chips, and trail mix--contain sulfur-based preservatives."*

I'm not sure that's such a good thing. Maybe I don't have to grow all my own food, but I can try to buy from local growers and only buy what I can use before it spoils, so that I don't have to rely on preservatives to keep my food "fresh." Is it really that fresh tasting and looking anyway?

How many food additives and preservatives do you consume in a day?

Go ahead – check the ingredients lists for the majority of food packages in your pantry and make a list of all the preservatives or additives.

It's difficult to know the difference between what's an additive and preservative, and it doesn't really matter, *it's in there!* You'll know one when you see it. Sometimes ingredients say what they're in there for, others are just the ones you can't pronounce, and sound like a chemical, are abbreviated (BHA) and some even have numbers.

Preservatives and Additives are everywhere in our food supply and some are dangerous, especially to little bodies (maybe the ones who ingest them the most). Food additives can affect certain behaviors, which can lead to attention-deficit hyperactivity disorder (ADHD). The behaviors caused by this disorder can seriously impact children's educational development.

I know several children who suffer from ADHD and their parents notice a huge difference in their behavior when they limit or remove some of the red and yellow food colorings from their children's diet. If you know a child with attention challenges or is hyper or wired, try to eliminate food colorings and see if you notice a difference.

Another reason I avoid food colorings is an example from my stepdad who's an avid feeder of hummingbirds. He's in his late 70's and we don't always agree about food supply issues, although he's starting to come around on many topics. One thing he is sure of is that his hummingbirds will not touch the feeder if he tries to trick them with red food coloring instead of actual grenadine (which gets its red color from pomegranates). The hummingbirds are smart and know the difference. As for food colorings and pesticides, if the bugs & birds don't want to eat it, neither do I!

Artificial colorings and preservatives are not only found in candy, they can be found in breakfast cereals, soft drinks, juices and other processed foods, including vitamins, toothpaste and over-the-counter medications.

Organics vs. Conventional

If organic farming is the natural way, shouldn't organic produce just be called "produce" and make the pesticide-laden stuff take the burden of an adjective? ~ Ymber Delecto

Organic

According to the USDA website, Certified Organic refers to *"a product that has been produced in accordance with specific regulations and that have been inspected and approved by an accredited certifying agent."* The USDA Federal Rule governing organic certification requires that an organic production system is managed *"to respond to site-specific conditions by integrating cultural, biological, and mechanical practices that foster cycling of resources, promote ecological balance, and conserve biodiversity."*

What percent of your diet is certified organic?

Conventional

Conventional Agriculture, according to the USDA's website is *"an industrialized agricultural system characterized by mechanization, monocultures, and the use of synthetic inputs such as chemical fertilizers and pesticides, with an emphasis on maximizing productivity and profitability."* Industrialized agriculture has become "conventional" only within the last 60 or so years (since World War II).

> ➤ **Genetically Modified Organisms (GMO's):**
Today, it seems you can't get away from genetically modified foods, because, according to Cornell University scientists, more than 60% of the food in U.S. grocery stores contains at least some small quantity of genetically altered crops. The corn and soybeans used in many processed foods are the most commonly genetically modified crops. The FDA is not required to routinely test GM foods for safety, and manufacturers aren't required to label foods as GM.

GM farming is considered safe for consumption by the FDA, but long-term effects are currently unknown. Commercial farmers, especially in the U.S., use genetic modification to alter crops for many reasons, such as producing greater quantities of a product, or to build resistance to pests or drought, or to "boost" its nutritional content. For example, genetic engineering allows for tomatoes to be grown with higher amounts of lycopene (a cancer preventing phytonutrient in the red pigment).

Today, we don't know exactly how safe GM foods are; some argue that the United States is dominating the world food market with their GM crops. There is some concern that altering the genetic makeup of food may be a cause for allergenic and/or antibiotic properties in foods, which could be dangerous.

> **Hormones and Antibiotics:**

When animals were taken out of pastures and put into prisons (inside pens or cages), they developed terrible diseases. To counter all the diseases from the dark, tight, unsanitary living spaces, the animals were given **antibiotics,** to which they grew resistant. Now what to do? Add more chemicals to counter that, and so on, for decades. Fast forward a few generations in the cycle and you have the industrialized meat market.

The human system was not designed for the industrial food chain!

For generations, the agro-meat business has been growing and expanding their huge, dark dungeons. The quarters are disgusting, but hamburgers are in high demand. Some of the big chains have sold so many hamburgers, I think they lost count! Somewhere along the way, the animals became so unhealthy that they needed something to "beef" them up. What to do? How about injecting them with **growth hormones**? OH BOY!!! Now the cows are fattening up and producing more than ever! Oh yay; more milk and meat to sell per cow! Now what? Give 'em some more of those "growth enhancers!"

Pesticides, herbicides and growth hormones are known as "unintentional contaminants," they "bioaccumulate" which means they build up in the organism consuming them. Because our bodies are not designed to ingest them and don't know what else to do with them, our sweet, wonderful bodies just absorb them and they build up and eventually cause disease.

All we have to do is fast forward a few more generations and we will have a very sick society. There's no wonder Americans have more disease today than ever! For more information about this topic visit www.pbs.org/tradescerets/.

> **Nitrites/ Nitrates**

Sodium nitrite is a simple salt used in manufacturing most *All-American* meat products, such as bacon, ham, hot dogs, and cold cuts. Nitrites have had a long and sordid past and are still in our food supply. Part of the debate is perhaps because some say they're a food coloring agent, so should be regulated by the Food and Drug Administration (FDA), while others say that it is a preservative and some of the meats to which they are added, like hot dogs, are not always cooked prior to eating, so they are necessary to keep them preserved. Somehow, they are still a significant part of the mainstream food supply, even though, in 1956, it was shown that nitrite could combine with nitrogen-containing amnio acids to form nitroamines, a powerful carcinogen in animals. Only traces of these nitroamines are found in cured meats, but they can be formed by cooking them. They can also be formed in the human digestive tract. The human body can even form nitroamines from nitrates which are found in vegetables grown with high-nitrate fertilizer (many of which are used in non-organic farming practices). There are many ways we can be accumulating nitroamines in our bodies and the combinations are highly carcinogenic and can be lethal for humans.

An MIT study in 1978 found that nitrites themselves could be a carcinogen; they produced cancer of the lymph system in rats. Based on the findings, the USDA ordered meat processors, over a period of several years, to decrease residual nitrite levels from an average of 200 parts per million to 40. Based on the Food Additives and Color Additives Amendments we just learned about, if these products were found to cause cancer in rats, why are they still in the food supply? Because a review of the MIT study in 1980 found some flaws with their diagnosis of lymphatic cancer, the FDA decided to take no further action. Who performed the review and why? It's up to the manufacturer to prove safety, the FDA has no requirements to seek further action, or more studies. Performing studies like these are very time and money consuming for universities and consumer groups. Big agribusiness corporations have a lot of money to lobby and fight testing, or find minute flaws that deem a study irrelevant.

> It seems like pesticides and potentially harmful chemicals are treated like criminals in our judicial system – they are innocent until proven guilty. Shouldn't it be the other way around?

What can you do about it? Vote with your dollars! As a single mom, I have a tight grocery budget, but the one thing I insist on is not purchasing foods with nitrates or nitrites. I purchase uncured bacon, lunch meats and hot dogs (my son doesn't even like hot dogs, but sometimes I still do).

> **Pesticides**

According to the United States Environmental Protection Agency (EPA), a pesticide is any substance or mixture of substances intended for:

- preventing
- destroying
- repelling
- mitigating any pest

Insecticides are pesticides. The term pesticide also applies to herbicides, fungicides, and many other substances used to control pests. In fact, herbicides are the most commonly used pesticide in the U.S. A pesticide is also any substance or "mixture of substances intended for use as a plant regulator, defoliant, or desiccant."

Pesticides were created after World War II using leftover chemical agents and ammunition, DDT and BHC were among the first pesticides to be used, and they quickly began to be widely used. Eventually they were discovered to be harmful to the environment and the animals and humans within it. Their liberal use made many pests and bacteria genetically resistant, non-target plants and animals became harmed, and pesticide residues were appearing in unexpected places.

As a result of pesticide toxicity, pesticide usage has been more scrutinized and requires more testing. But still, their extensive use in the US. and many other countries is alarming. Many of the common pesticides used today are derivatives of those original poisons (gun powder anyone?) and are still made by the same powerful companies (companies whose board members have been the top executives of the United States government).

Pesticide usage is widespread in the U.S. They are used on hundreds of thousands of farms and in millions of households. Agriculture is responsible for about 75 percent of all pesticide usage, but 85 percent of households in the U.S. have at least one pesticide in them, and 63 percent have up to five!

The pesticides used in home landscaping and gardening and in agriculture and agro-business are toxic to the planet and our bodies and many of them are known carcinogens! When used, only about 10% of the pesticide actually goes towards the target product, the rest runs off into surface and ground water.

Like most toxins, pesticides bio-accumulate. That is why pesticides are found in the highest concentration in animal based products! The bigger the animal or fish, or the higher up the food chain, the more toxins have bio-accumulated. WOW! Some of our bodies probably have pretty high concentrations of toxins, pesticides and growth hormones too.

What percent of the food you consume in a day is conventionally grown?

So, what's the best bet for your body? Conventional or Organic?

Processed foods are processed, so their natural state has been altered. Some foods are further from nature than others. There are many reasons, as we've seen, for foods to be altered from their natural state, including convenience, food safety, taste, and longer shelf life.

Processing as we know it today can deplete the naturally occurring nutrients in foods, like antioxidants, phytonutrients, vitamins, and minerals. Processing can try to replace some of these, but not all, and a processed product is no longer natural and ultimately not as good for us. The synthetic nutrients, like vitamins and minerals that some manufacturers add to some foods, aren't as powerful as the original or naturally occurring nutrients. Please note, however, that some nutrients added to processed foods can have great health benefits, like iron fortified cereal.

There are some healthy examples of processed foods, such as fruits and vegetables that are flash frozen at their peak of freshness. These sometimes have more nutritional value than fresh varieties that have traveled over long distances and were picked when not yet ripe. Some flash frozen fish and meat products are also good choices because they are extremely fresh-tasting.

Some less healthy examples of processed foods are highly processed snack and junk foods that have little or no nutritional value and are high in calories and/or fat, sugar and salt, like cookies, sweets, crackers and chips.

With all the unknown health and environmental risks associated to GM foods and additives, it's best to stick to whole foods. By following a so-called whole foods diet, it is possible to avoid many GM foods and additives. Not very many raw fruits and vegetables are genetically modified. What you may want to question and stay away from are the non-organic, processed foods made with corn or soy.

As for me and my family, when it comes to the safety of my food supply; I'll stick with Mother Nature and try to avoid chemical and over-processed foods. I purchase certified organic products, especially animal-based products, whenever possible. I also grow my own organic vegetables, which is a wonderful way to eat. Many cities have Pea Patch or community garden programs for residents that don't have their own garden space.

In high school and much of college I worked in either a health food store or food cooperative, so I'm lucky that I was drawn at an early age to natural foods. I also love the human body. That's why I studied nutrition in the first place, along with thinking it would make me useful in the Peace Corps. I care about what goes into my mouth, my children's mouths, and into the environment we live in, so that's why I choose my foods with purpose and taste in mind. Besides if a bug doesn't want to eat a product with those chemicals on it, why would I?

Taste Test

Non-conventional foods do taste better! Try a taste test for yourself! After years of trying to get my mom to buy organics, she finally came to me and said that she broke down and bought organic apples and they were so delicious they reminded her of *"the apples when I was a kid."* She had actually stopped liking or even buying apples, but now that she buys organic apples, she enjoys them again! I think you'll find you can tell a difference from conventionally grown and organic products.

How to have your own taste test:
1) Purchase some conventional and organic produce, such as apples and carrots.
2) Before you begin, hold each item and look it over for color, spots, feel.
3) Close your eyes and breathe in the scent of the fruit or vegetable.
4) Now, wash each one and prepare it how you like. Raw slices work well.
5) Hold each piece and breathe in its essence.
6) Take a bite.
7) How does each one taste?
8) How does it feel on your tongue? As you swallow it?

9) Does either of them taste better?
10) Could you feel that each one was a cellular organism, one that lived and breathed?

Not only does most organic produce taste better, but organic meats (raised without hormones and fed a plant-based, organic diet) taste better, too. Since pesticides and hormones bio-accumulate, the meat products develop a different taste. Cows and chickens that were created to eat plant-based, vegetarian products that are fed animal by-products have a distinctive flavor. I've even been told by some friends that his/her lover, who converted to an organic, plant-based diet "tasted" better. Even our own natural muskiness can be affected by the foods we eat!

Some people may argue that buying organic or shopping at natural food stores is more expensive, All I can say is you have to decide if it's worth it to you. Cost should not take precedence over protecting our good health. Would you rather continue to eat a multitude of chemicals with your food? Even my brother, who can afford to buy any kind of food he wants, is slow to change and mentions the cost. My response to him is "you're worth it and so are your kids!" I struggle with economy and the cost of food is a huge concern for me, so I do my best to purchase what feels right for me. Whatever your choice, enjoy the foods you eat.

Food Safety

Food Safety could very easily and rightfully be an entire chapter on its own, but since this isn't a textbook, I have no intention of delving too deep into the subject. We'll just cover the basics…

Danger Zone: 40° - 140°
This is the temperature range where bacteria grow most rapidly. Harmful bacteria can double in number in as few as 20 minutes. This is why it is recommended that you not leave perishable food out of the fridge for more than two hours. If a food is already above 90° you shouldn't leave it out for more than one hour. If a product has been left in the danger zone and grows bacteria, many of those bacteria are heat resistant, meaning heating the food will not kill the harmful bacteria and you can still get sick, very sick. When in doubt, throw it out!

Safe minimum cooking temperatures:
Beef, veal and lamb steaks, roasts and chops = 145 °F
Pork, ground beef, veal and lamb = 160 °F
Poultry (and leftovers) = 165 °F throughout

When cooking meat and poultry, your oven temperature should never be below 325°.

Defrosting:
One of my former colleagues tells this story *"I suggested to my class that they could defrost their meat in the microwave and one of my participants came back to me and told me her whole family got sick. I asked her how she defrosted it and she said 'I put it in the microwave like you said'."* The woman had put the meat in the microwave in the morning and left it there all day thinking that somehow it was safe from attracting bacteria.

Be careful when defrosting. Try to leave yourself a day or two for your product to defrost in a refrigerator that is between 34 ° - 40°. It should be put on the lowest possible shelf, sealed, and on a plate or pan to make sure none of the juices escape and contaminate other products. If you must defrost an item in a hurry, the microwave has a defrost function, however, sometimes it may actually cook part of the meat.

Expiration Dates:
There has been some controversy lately regarding convenient marts selling products that are well passed the selling date. Be sure to check those dates when purchasing perishable items.

- **Best if used by and use-by date**: This is the date by which the product should maintain maximum freshness, flavor and texture. It is not a purchase-by or safety date of any type; it just means that past this date, although it may still be edible, the product begins to deteriorate.
- **Expiration date**: Do not use a product past this date, it is no longer fresh and may be hazardous to your health after this date.
- **Sell-by or pull-by date**: The manufacturer uses this date to inform grocers when to remove their product from the shelves. It doesn't mean it's not safe for home use beyond this date. For example, milk often has a sell-by date, but the milk usually doesn't spoil for at least a week beyond that date, if refrigerated.
- **Guaranteed fresh**: This date is often used for perishable baked goods. Again, an item may still be edible but it may not be fresh.

- **Packed on**: This is the date the item was packaged, and usually it is used on canned and boxed goods. Generally this date is an encrypted code, and is not always easy to decipher. It may be coded by month (M), day (D), and year (Y), such as YYMMDD or MMDDYY.

School Lunch

Even if you do not have children who eat at school or will eventually eat at school, please read this section on school lunch, because **children are our future**. While children are at school, it would seem logical that they be sparred from being served substances that are harmful to their growth, their development, and their environment. Not so! School lunches in the USA are appalling. When I was young, my grandmother (who died in 1980) worked at a school cafeteria and she was so proud of her job! She felt honored to be able to prepare and serve good food for the children of her community. Those days are not totally over for the public schools of America, though we have strayed far, far away since then.

As a community health educator I've been to many public schools to give workshops and trainings and I've talked to a lot of parents and teachers and have seen some horrifying menus. Many of the menus I've seen are not much different from the cafeteria in the movie *Super Size Me*. If you haven't seen the movie, I highly recommend it: it's very entertaining and educational. The main utensil a school "chef" used was a box cutter to open boxes of frozen food. Boxes of pre-packaged, processed burritos, hot dogs, and pizzas have replaced grandmas like mine in the lunch line. They are cheap and easy to make and prepare, and yield a high profit margin for the manufacturer, (not necessarily the school). The chefs at box cutter schools assured me that the menus meet federal school lunch standards. Don't the federal standards account for the absurdly high sodium, fat and sugar contents of the food being served? No, those substances do not have a Daily Reference Intake (RDI), therefore no federal standards.

It doesn't make sense to me that children may take a health class in the same environment where they are being sold unhealthy food for lunch. School is where children go to learn, isn't that a mixed message?

The Center for Science in the Public Interest (CSPI) recently graded school lunches in the U.S. and most states got poor – if not failing – grades on school food policies. Could this be why over the past 20 years, obesity rates of American children and teenagers have tripled? Or is it because only 2 percent of them eat a diet that meets USDA standards?

20 years of changes for food and schools in America:
- ✓ Big corporations were able to buy their way onto campuses, even elementary schools, and they gave big money and made big money and also gained consumers for life through market branding. (For more information on marketing visit Chapter 4, Media Madness). Thankfully, this behavior is coming into check and with more people speaking up, we'll see more healthy choices available in schools.
- ✓ Corn syrup started to dominate the food supply because of an over-production of corn. What to do with too much corn? Turn it into sweet, sweet syrup and add it to everything from bread to water and sell it for a huge profit.
- ✓ Portion sizes grew dramatically. How big were bagels 20 years ago? How big is a bagel today? Take the Portion Distortion quiz, information in Chapter 6.

The CSPI recently gave high marks to Kentucky and Oregon for their school food policies. Although CSPI reports that 2/3 of our states have weak, if any, nutritional standards and fail to limit junk food and soda sales on campus. Only ten states address trans-fats (a manufactured fat that is dangerous to the human system, more about fats in the next chapter). Just five states limit sodium in school foods. It's no wonder my eyes popped out of my head when I saw the sodium content of one local school's menu.

The USDA set goals for all schools to have policies and many school boards have slowly been working on them. At one meeting I attended, in the attempt to help the board make better choices for the schools, I was told that as an outsider (although a health professional who lived and worked in the community), I was not allowed to speak at the meetings. Yes, I had to remain silent! I must report that I was dismayed by the results of that school's policies. It's shocking how much adults will put children at risk in order for them not to have to change their own habits. The teachers did not want to ban soda sales because they liked to stock their refrigerator in the staff room with sodas and thought that it would be a contradiction if they didn't let the kids have it, too. It's honorable that they didn't want to be hypocritical; however, it's pathetic that they made their choices based on their own wants, not the physiological needs of their growing, learning students.

> **It seems to me that the decisions about our food supply are being made without the public interest in mind. People are making choices for others based on their own wants and desires. Sadly, many of the decisions made in countries like mine are based on the profits (and desires) of very few individuals and corporations.**

School lunches have definitely taken a downturn from the 70's when my grandma worked in a cafeteria. However, there are some schools, and even entire districts, making wonderful advancements in the ways meals are served at schools. I've seen schools run side-by-side, where one school's lunches come from boxes and one has fresh produce and dairy, and the meats come from local farms. A lot depends on the person in charge of the lunches at your school (or district). It also depends on parents, caregivers and teachers getting involved and insisting on better meals at schools.

What are the school lunches like in your community?

If you've got a child in your life that goes to school and you don't know where their lunches come from, I encourage you to find out. If you're not satisfied with what is being offered, get involved!!! Talk to the Superintendent, go to the Board. Children deserve fresh, healthy food!

> **Some parents and caregivers may not have had education themselves and don't know the best food choices to make at home, so they may look to the school and ask themselves** *"what do they provide? I'll serve that too."* **It is crucial that schools be the ones teaching our children and families the right food choices!**

With all the cuts in education over the last several years, schools have taken a hit and some are depending more than ever on corporate contracts. There are better choices for vending machines as well. Many health food vendors carry bottled water, fruit juice and rice milk in addition to cow's milk. Some schools blame low sales or student revolt for not converting to healthier choices, but most schools who have made the change to healthy vending are happier for it! Studies reflect that there may be an initial downturn in sales, but it quickly picks up pace and exceeds junk food sales. When schools serve attractive raw produce like baby carrots, celery and fresh pineapple, children start to enjoy fruits and vegetables more and regularly include them in their diets.

If we're going to make our country healthy again and reverse the growing rates of obesity and diabetes, we have to start with the children. Today's children are among the first in the history of the United States to have a lower life expectancy than their parents! The best place to start helping children be healthier is in our schools. Let's work together to make schools healthy again! Let's do it for today's children, tomorrow's children and the lunch ladies of yesteryear!

Mother Nature knows best; fuel your system with her foods first!

NOTES

NOTES

Chapter Three

Supermarket Savvy

As for butter versus margarine, I trust cows more than chemists ~
Joan Gussow

Since we're talking about our bodies and the food (fuel) we give it, we might as well talk about the supermarket, grocery store, or whatever you call the place where you buy groceries. Either way, all of us go there at some time or another, and if you prepare the meals in your household, you probably go there even more than you'd like. Let's take a walk through the average supermarket and look at what's inside, which is a great step in the right direction for making the best food choices.

Read Thy Label

The Nutrition Facts Panel is the most important part of the packaged food you purchase, please, please, pretty please, read your labels!

Before we get started on the label, you'll need a couple of food packages with nutrition labels so you can follow along. Check your cupboards for some packages. Good examples might be bread, cereal, and a convenience item like boxed rice, or a frozen meal.

Ingredients

Of utmost importance on your package label is the ingredient list. Scrutinize your ingredient list. **Can you identify every item?** Chances are if you have never heard of an ingredient, you can't pronounce it, or it's more than 10 letters long, you probably don't want to eat it! Your vehicle (body) was not designed for those chemicals. But, there are certain products your vehicle was designed for: fresh fruits and vegetables, whole grains, nuts, seeds and beans, and local, natural meat products.

.

Nutrition Facts

Serving Size

Servings Per Container

Amount per serving

Calories   Calories from Fat

% Daily Value

Total Fat

  Saturated Fat

  Trans Fat

Cholesterol

Sodium

Total Carbohydrate

  Dietary Fiber

  Sugars

Protein

Vitamin A   Vitamin C

Calcium   Iron

Percent Daily Value (DV)
This is what percent of the nutrient a particular food item has based on an average caloric intake.

Daily Reference Intake (DRI) –
These reference values are there to help individuals optimize their health, prevent disease, and avoid consuming too much of any one nutrient. DRI's combine four reference values, 2 of which are **Daily Recommended Allowance** (RDA), or daily dietary nutrient Intake sufficient to meet ~ 98% of healthy people and **Tolerable Uptake Levels** (UL), highest level that is likely not to pose a risk to the general population.

Fat – Total fats should be at least 20% and not more than 35% of total calories. Since we really don't need that much added fat in our diets for our bodies to function properly (about a tablespoon will do), stick with the smallest amount you can. The best fats come from fish, nuts, avocados, olives, vegetable oils, and butter. Saturated fats should be no more than 10% of total fat intake.

Fats are sometimes broken down into their parts:

❖ **Cholesterol** – Found only in animal tissue. Liver and egg yolks are found to have high amounts of cholesterol. Lipids are transported through our bodies covered in a protein coat called lipoprotein, and the amounts of these lipoproteins in our blood help to determine the state of our health. LDL (low density lipoprotein) has less protein and more cholesterol, which increases the risk for developing coronary heart disease. High Density Lipoproteins (HDL) has higher protein levels relative to the cholesterol. The lower the density of lipoprotein, the more fat there is, and the more damaging it is for the cardiovascular system. If you consume too much cholesterol, you increase your LDL levels and cause strain on your heart.

❖ **Saturated Fat** – Think of saturated fats as soaked sponges. From a chemical view, all the carbon atoms are bonded with hydrogen, which means that once they are saturated, they cannot bond with any other molecule. Saturated fats come mostly from animal fats and dairy products, and they are also found in any fat (oil) that remains solid at room temperature, such as the tropical oils (coconut and palm) and shortening. Limit saturated fat to 10% (or about 16 grams per day for most people). Not all saturated fats are created equal; some have longer chains than others, and the longer the chain, the worse it is. Butter, coconut and palm kernel oils have short and medium chains, thus, they are not responsible for raising cholesterol levels or causing heart disease. Long-chain saturates are the "bad" fats: they're responsible for raising LDL and lowering HDL and are found in red meats like beef, veal, lamb, and pork. Hydrogenation creates long-chain saturates and virtually turns the fatty acids into toxin (see Trans Fat below).

❖ **Trans Fat** – This is a chemical fat made in a laboratory. It is plant-based unsaturated oil that has been **trans**formed into a saturated fat. Once again, it is another manufactured, processed food product that our bodies were not designed to ingest or digest and so our bodies don't know what to do with it. It is even more harmful than lard (animal fat) because it is not natural.

Processed food products are loaded with trans fatty acids because it gives them a longer shelf life.

o   Trans fat can be found in: cookies, chips, fried food, cakes, breads, candy, margarine, salad dressings, and baked products. Usually the ingredient list will say "hydrolyzed" or "hydrogenated", that's how you'll know the fat or oil has been transformed.

o   0 grams = does not mean zero. The American Heart Association recommends we eat no more than 2 grams of trans fats a day. The USDA has approved that if a product contains less than .5 (or ½) grams of trans fat it can claim 0 grams. However, eating many products with ½ a gram of trans fat could add up without your knowing it. Check your labels! If a product says it has 0 grams trans fat, but it is a highly processed boxed product like cookies, crackers, margarine, or coffee creamer, check the ingredient list, and if it says hydrogenated oil, it has some trans fat in it.

o   If you don't want to read all of your labels, most Organic food manufacturers voluntarily do not use hydrogenated oils, so organics are usually a better choice. If in doubt, read it out.

❖   **Fried Foods** – While we're on the topic of fat, we might as well discuss fried foods. Think about your car. Would you purposefully put bad, already used, burned up oil in your car? Probably not. Why is that? Do you think twice before putting fried foods into your body, your vehicle? When we ingest fried foods, we're putting bad, used up oil into our machines. The oil used in frying reaches extreme temperatures of up to 500°, so that oil is burned up. When vegetable oil is heated at high temperatures it rapidly oxidizes and quickly becomes rancid. Have you heard the term "energy is never created or destroyed?" All that heat (energy) has now been transferred into the food that was fried. No wonder so many people complain of heartburn after eating a big, greasy, fried meal. There is also evidence that this heated, oxidized oil increases free radical damage to our cells, therefore causing more cancer risk. Don't get me wrong, I love French fries, and I'm also a sucker for Buffalo wings, which are deep fried. However, I only eat this stuff every once in a while.

In one of my nutrition education classes, we had an exercise about fast food. I would set up different 'fast food restaurants,' around the room using fake, cardboard food. The restaurants ranged from Pizza Hut to Burger King, KFC, etc... The participants browsed through them and picked out a lunch. We would join together and the participants wrote down the nutritional content of their choice, then we would review it and pick out better choices for them to make.   One woman was very surprised when she was told that the hamburger was a better choice than the chicken sandwich she chose.   The chicken sandwich had almost twice the amount of fat because it was fried and therefore not a good choice, especially when coupled with French fries.

The Good Fats

The majority of the good fats will be liquid at room temperature. Many of these fatty acids have protective qualities for our bodies, as well as antioxidant properties. Generally, the more liquid the fat, the better it is for you. However, there is one saturated fat that makes it on the list of good fats and that's coconut oil. It has medium chain triglycerides (the chemical form of fat), which makes it move through the body easier than other saturated fats with long, complicated chains.

Monounsaturated Fatty Acids – This means that one carbon atom is free of hydrogen, thus, it is not saturated. They remain liquid at room temperature, but solidify in colder temperatures. Monounsaturated fats are mostly found in canola, olive and peanut oils. Canola oil is genetically modified rapeseed oil and not the most highly recommended oil. Peanut oil is heavily refined. Extra-virgin olive oil is the most highly recommended oil to use for cooking; it cannot be used for stir-frying (at high temperatures), because it has a low melting point, which means it will scorch or burn at a lower temperature than most other oils. Light olive oil has been processed to remove many of the good fats and is not recommended.
Polyunsaturated Fatty Acids – More than one carbon atom is free of hydrogen. These are mostly found in corn, safflower, flaxseed, sesame, soybean, macadamia, sunflower and some fish oils. They are highly recommended because they actually lower both LDL and HDL cholesterol. However, safflower and corn oil are not recommended as highly because of their essential fatty acid ratio (see below).

Essential Fatty Acids (EFA's)
These are unsaturated fats that the body cannot make on its own, like the essential amino acids, so they must be consumed through the diet. EFA's are used in our body to rebuild and make new cells, regulate body functions, like immune response, blood clot formation, inflammation, and injury response.
Omega-3 (O-3) Essential Fatty Acid (alpha-linolenic acid) – found in fish (SALMON), fish oil, flax seeds (ground into a meal) and flax oil, wheat germ, walnuts, soy, pecans and pumpkin seeds.
Omega-6 (O-6) Essential Fatty Acid (linoleic acid) – raw nuts, seeds, legumes, corn, corn oil and safflower oil.

- Omega 3 vs. Omega 6 ratio: These two fats fight with each other to gain access into the membranes around each cell of our bodies. They each play different roles once they get into the cells. About 100 years ago, when we ate only free range, "organic" animal foodstuff; these products were enough to satisfy our body's needs for omega-3. Fast forward to today and a big change in our body's EFA balance. Because the meat we consume is industrialized, the animals themselves are consuming too much omega-6 (cows a hundred years ago did not eat corn!), their meat contains high levels of omega-6, so we eat too much O-6 ourselves. Omega-3 (O-3) is being edged out of our diets.
- Low Omega-3, High Omega-6: The result of not enough O-3 is that O-3 actually builds the cell membrane, namely around the brain and heart. Are you following me? Low O-3 can lead to stroke, heart attack, and insulin resistance among other serious diseases. O-3 is also responsible for keeping a nice fatty brain, and research shows that brains lacking in strong membranes are more prone to hostility, possibly depression, and even Alzheimer's disease. Because of the skewed ratio in EFA's it is highly recommended we eat more O-3. Salmon is the best source; you should eat it two to three times a week for optimum absorption. Another good way to include more O-3 is adding ground flax meal or wheat germ to yogurt and cereals. Fish oil or flax oil supplements are another idea; you may want to check with your health care professional before you take any supplements.
- Wild salmon eat algae and seaweed which boosts their O-3 levels. Farm raised salmon do not have the levels of

O-3 that wild fish do, that's one reason why eating wild caught fish is the better choice. Like other farmed raised animals, farmed fish also have more antibiotics and hormones than are found in wild fish.

Butter vs. the other stuff

In my opinion, the quote at the beginning of the chapter sums it up – butter is better! Yes, butter is a saturated fat and we're supposed to limit those, but it's still far better than the hydrogenated, trans fats found in imitation/ margarine type products. Here is a list of reasons why butter is better:
* Butter has lecithin which helps our bodies break down cholesterol.
* Butter is a good source of Vitamin A, E and Selenium which are powerful antioxidants.
* The saturated fats in butter are short and medium chain fatty acids which have protective qualities, unlike the long chain fatty acids in red meat (and many margarine products).
* Butter has conjugated linolenic acid
* Butter is only 80% fat, margarine is 100% fat!

** If you must use margarine because your doctor highly recommends it, tub margarine is better than cube and be sure the trans fat and saturated fat content are no more than 2 grams.

Total Carbs – How many carbohydrates are in the product?

Carbohydrates are sometimes broken down into their parts:
* **Sugar –** *Why is there no DRA for sugar in the US?* Since we don't have one in the U.S, let's go with what the Canadians say – 40 grams a day! Unlike Canada and the UK, the US will not give a recommended daily amount for sugar. There is a limit and should be; however, I think there is not one because sugar (namely high fructose corn syrup) is BIG BUSINESS in America and BIG BUSINESS has a lot of influence in a capitalized market!
* If a product is more than 50% sugar, you probably should avoid it, because that product is mostly sugar. To find what percent of sugar is in your product, take the **total sugars and divide that by the total calories**. You may be surprised to find that some of your favorite items and even "healthy" ones have a lot of sugar.

o   Do your math to determine what % of sugar is in a product: we learned in Chapter Two that sugar has 4 calories per gram.
o   Take the grams of sugar in the product and multiply it by 4, divide that by the total calories = now move decimal place over 2 places = % sugar.
  ▪   So if a product has 120 calories and 29 grams of sugar =
    •   29*4/120 = 96% sugar!

PLEASE LIMIT your total daily sugar content to 40 grams!
Every 4 grams of sugar = one teaspoon

* Thankfully, in the August 25, 2009 edition of the Wall Street Journal, there is an article about the American Heart Association's recommendation to consume no more than 100 grams of sugar a day! We're getting somewhere...

❖ **Fiber** – Something most Americans could use more of in their daily diet is fiber.
Fiber helps:
  •   With weight loss
  •   Lower cholesterol
  •   Control blood sugar
  •   Ease bowel movements and keep digestive tract on track.

  ➤   **Some tips for getting more fiber:**
  ✓   Eat brown rice and whole grains instead of white rice, bread, and pasta
  ✓   Choose whole grain cereals for breakfast
  ✓   Have plenty of precut raw vegetables to snack on instead of chips, crackers, or chocolate bars
  ✓   Substitute beans and legumes for meat two to three times per week. Put them in soups, chili, rice dishes, salads, etc.
  ✓   Eat whole fruits instead of drinking fruit juices (if you're going to drink juice, make sure it says "**100% fruit juice**". If the package says "real juice", or just "fruit juice," it is not really juice, but colored, flavored sugar (or corn syrup).

✓ Experiment with international dishes that use whole grains and legumes as part of the main meal. For example Indian dahls with pilau rice or in Middle Eastern salads like tabbouleh, or falafel.

Protein – How much protein is in the product? As we discussed in the last chapter, most adults have no problem meeting their protein requirements. It's how much we get and when we eat it that helps us stay strong and vital throughout the day. A small amount of protein rich foods at breakfast and lunch is recommended. Also, if you do extensive exercise it's a good idea to eat some protein before, and especially after, a workout. For more information about pre and post workout snacks, visit Chapter 5. See Chapter 2 for a list of protein rich foods.

Miles of Aisles

Most markets are laid out in convenient aisles with the frozen or convenience stuff in the middle, the vegetables and breads on the ends, and dairy in the back.

Foods along the outside edge of the store are the most whole, natural choices; they are mostly the unboxed items. If you stick to doing most of your shopping along the outside perimeter of the store, you'll be purchasing mostly fresh, unprocessed foods. Go to the fish department, butcher, dairy case, fresh bakery. The closer to the middle of the store, the more processed the foods are.

Foods are put on the shelves with specific tactics: food manufacturers pay for their placements on the shelves. It doesn't matter what grocery store you're in, the food companies are buying prime shelf space, just like they buy prime time advertising spots on TV. The more the company pays, the closer to eye level their products are placed. Wherever a product is placed on the shelf is no indication of how good it is for you, or how healthy it is. More likely, the healthiest stuff is on the bottom shelf.

The one exception is the stores that have specific "health food" sections. Here you might find good foods at eye level or down by your feet. These companies are still paying for prime space and some so-called health foods are still highly processed and not the best choices.

Store perimeter:

Produce section: Notice the colors and shapes of all the fruits and vegetables. Shop with variety in mind and eat the rainbow! Instead of just broccoli, eat cauliflower, cabbage, Brussels sprouts, and bok choy. A sweet potato cooks up just like a regular potato and offers different phyto nutrients: in fact, each color has different antioxidants. That's why we say 'Eat the Rainbow.' Yum! Same goes for fruit. Mix it up, try something new. Frozen berries thaw out very well and are great choices! Always choose the fruits and vegetables that look freshest. Get to know your Produce Manager, because he's there to help and you can always ask him if he's got a better looking bunch of whatever you're after in the back.

Most supermarkets now have organic food sections. We cover organics in greater detail in the Food Is Fuel chapter; however, it's important to mention them here, too. I (along with many other health professionals) am an advocate of organic farming practices because it is a more sustainable form of agriculture for our planet. There is evidence that farm workers who apply chemicals to crops have increased risk of cancer because of the high rate of chemical contamination in their bodies.

> **On a personal note, when I worked for the Migrant Head Start program in Central California, I counseled parents of preschoolers on nutrition. All of the parents were migrant farm workers, mostly from Mexico. I could always tell when one of the parents was a pesticide sprayer, because the fumes on their clothes and bodies were so strong that on a number of occasions I experienced coughing fits, so much so that I had to open my office door. I was already convinced about the benefits of organics, but that reassured me that I did not want to eat food with those chemicals if I could avoid it.**

If you're concerned about pesticide residue on your non-organic produce, wash it with a dilute solution of dish soap and then rinse it under cool water for at least a minute. Pesticides are designed to attach to fat molecules and kill pests. Washing them with soap, which is a fat, causes the chemicals to attach to the soap and rinse off the produce. You should always rinse your produce anyway, even products you're going to peel or cut. When cutting or peeling an item, the residue, or even dirt, from others who have handled the produce can cross into the fruit inside: this is called cross-contamination.

Brix scores: Organic farmers tend to use high-brix farming practices. A high Brix score is produced by practices that make the fruits and vegetables have higher levels of sugar, as well as amino acids, oils, flavonoids, minerals, and other nutrients. This is why most people agree that many organic products taste better, as a higher Brix score means they are sweeter and full of other natural occurring flavor enhancers.

Of course, organics do tend to be more expensive and it's not always economical to purchase them. As a single mom, I watch my budget, but the items I insist on buying organic are the "dirty dozen." Each year the Environmental Working Group tests about 45 fruits and vegetables for pesticide residue, this produce is tested after it has been rinsed and peeled. The dirty dozen are the ones that have the most residues. Ironically these also tend to be the items I think simply taste better as organic.

Produce:	**Score:**
1. Peach	100 (highest pesticide load)
2. Apple	93
3. Sweet Bell Pepper	83
4. Celery	82
5. Nectarine	81
6. Strawberries	80
7. Cherries	73
8. Kale	69
9. Lettuce	67
10. Grapes – Imported	66
11. Carrot	63
12. Pear	63

The "clean dozen" Are:
1. Onion
2. Avocado
3. Sweet corn
4. Pineapples
5. Mango
6. Asparagus
7. Sweet peas
8. Kiwi
9. Cabbage
10. Eggplant
11. Papaya
12. Watermelon

I accessed this above information from the Environmental Working Group's website (1/19/2010). You can download a printable, wallet-sized chart at: www.foodnews.org/walletguide.php. They also have an iPhone ap you can download.

Stock up on your fruit or veggies while they're fresh and in season and freeze them for later. They're easy to freeze, simply rinse them and drain them in a colander, place them in a single layer on a baking sheet and put the whole sheet in the freezer. When the produce is completely frozen, transfer them to a freezer bag and viola, you've got fresh frozen berries for your next smoothie, oatmeal, or yogurt.

Meat: The butcher and seafood sections are usually near the produce aisle. Again, the question of organics comes up. Since meat and dairy products are a rich source of fat in our diets, and so many of the contaminants in foods are fat soluble, I go organic when possible. Buying organic in this department also minimizes the amount of antibiotic residue we consume, which is a wise tactic for our future health and the health of our children.

Dairy:
Why is the dairy usually in the back of the store? The most common item we run out of is milk and the most common reason we're at the market is to "run in" for milk. If they put the dairy all the way in the back of the store, you'll have to walk past all those other items and chances are you're not walking out of there with just milk! Of course, the supermarket is there to sell you stuff and the more stuff they sell you, the more money they make!

Milk: Here we go again, to go organic or not to go organic? For all the reasons I've previously stated, yes, go organic if you can afford it. If not, choose the freshest most local products and enjoy. Besides organic, there are other choices as far as fat content. A good strategy is to go with the least fat content your taste buds can muster. Nonfat is the best choice, it reduces your intake of fat and cholesterol and leaves room in your diet for other fat containing products. If you just don't like the taste or consistency, 1% is great, or 2%.

The big problem with milk is lactose intolerance. This means a person lacks the enzymes to digest lactose, or milk sugar. Many people lose the ability to digest lactose as they age. However they don't lose it completely, so they can only handle it in small doses. If you think you do not tolerate lactose well because you get congested when you consume it, or you experience digestive problems like gas and bloating, see your doctor. But, also try consuming it in smaller amounts at a time. Trying less than one cup (8 ounces) at a time may help ease your symptoms. Goat's milk has less lactose than cow's milk, so that may be a good alternative, also. Many people who have trouble with milk can also consume cheese and yogurt without harm without a problem.

Yogurt: Beware of yogurt! Don't get me wrong, yogurt is a great food choice. It's got a fair amount of protein, is low in fat and has great bacterial cultures (called probiotics) which help maintain intestinal health. Watch out for the sugar content, though. Plain milk has about 12 grams of carbohydrate that come from the milk sugar or lactose, and it's a good carb. Read the label of plain yogurt and it's the same amount. Now, choose a flavored yogurt and the amount of carbohydrates and sugars rises up to the 20's and 30's. This means that the amount of sugars in the product has nearly doubled! Your best bet is to choose plain yogurt and sweeten it with fresh or frozen thawed fruit, honey, maple syrup, or agave syrup.

Cheese: Cheese is a great source of protein and calcium, but it is also high in fat. Regular cheddar cheese has about 7 grams of protein and 9 grams of fat per ounce (6 of which are saturated). It doesn't mean regular cheeses aren't good for you, it just means you should be mindful of how much you're eating to limit the amount of saturated fat you're getting.
Low-fat cheeses: Many light cheeses aren't very tasty, in my opinion. Some of them, however, are really good. Part-skim mozzarella and provolone cheese are delicious; they melt well and are great on sandwiches.

Eggs: These are usually in or near the dairy aisle, and again, boy are there a lot of choices! I like to go with the organic, vegetarian-fed eggs, but when I can't do that, I pick the ones that were raised in the state where I live. Omega-3 enhanced eggs are a good way to increase EFA's in your diet. The chickens themselves are fed flaxseed and have a slightly lower cholesterol level.

Bakery: The baked goods are usually along one of the four walls of the store. Many supermarkets are starting to bake and sell hearty rustic breads. These breads often have healthy ingredients like olives, walnuts and roasted garlic. There are some whole grain options, but usually they aren't 100% whole grain and many are purely refined. A good way to boost their nutritional value is to dip them in some extra virgin olive oil and balsamic vinegar, you can even add herbs like basil and rosemary or roasted garlic. Yum.

You hear a lot about the qualities of flax today, and many types of bread are adding whole flax to increase sales. The benefits of flax come from the ground product or oil, not the whole seed. If you're looking for a higher fiber product when purchasing bread, remember to read the label and take the 100% whole wheat bread. If it doesn't say 100%, it's not whole wheat and is simply white bread with a sugar, like high fructose corn syrup, added to make it brown.

Frozen Foods As we move to the center of the store, we find more of the processed products. However, the frozen section still has a lot of great choices. Frozen fruits and vegetables are healthy and nutritious alternatives to fresh as long as they aren't loaded with sauces. They are actually often even fresher than 'fresh' produce that has been sitting in your fridge wilting for a week or more.

A popular frozen product these days are the soy breakfast, deli and cheese products. As I mentioned in the beans section, beware of soy. Soy products that have been altered and transformed are not necessarily better for you than the real meat product that the soy product is pretending to be. There is a lot of research to support that soy products are unsafe, especially for young people. Before you make a habit of these tasty meat alternatives, do your research and determine if you're willing to take the risks.

Cereal: This is clearly a huge part of the American diet. You can tell because the cereal section usually takes up one whole aisle, if not two! The ones with the least amount of sugar are usually found on the bottom shelves. The candy coated cereals are at eye level. Thankfully, my son has only been minimally introduced to the sugary cereals and he doesn't care for them. Whew, that's one win in my house, but he sure has a sweet tooth for other items.

What are you eating cereal for, dessert or part of your nourishment? Many cereals have a lot of sugar, so just like with yogurt, determine how much sugar is in your cereal. Some of the whole grain cereal products that are all wheat have zero grams of sugar, if you compare them to other products, you'll see that any amount of sugar in other cereal products is added sugar. The one exception to this rule is if fruit is added, but this will account for a very small amount of sugar, since very little fruit is actually added to cereals. Keep in mind that every 4 grams of sugar equals one teaspoon of sugar!

Another thing to consider in your cereal is fiber and protein content. Looking at the all whole wheat cereal products or plain oatmeal, they contain about six grams of fiber and six grams of protein for one cup. That's a lot of nutrition with little calories. Compare that to your other choices, and you'll soon be able to tell which cereals are more processed (and more like candy) and which ones are providing substantial nutritional value.

I remember when I was a little girl, commercials for some of the sugary products used to show a bowl of cereal, a glass of orange juice, and milk. The announcer would say "part of a nutritious breakfast" to make you think it was healthy, when what was healthy was the other items, not the cereal. Today, I notice that these same products say "part of a good breakfast." They are no longer claiming they're part of a nutritious breakfast, but good breakfast. I guess they're telling the truth, because it tastes good, doesn't it?

Have you ever wondered why cereal is so expensive? It's because only five companies make about 85% of all the cereals on the market. This means no price competition, so branded cereals are priced much higher than it costs to produce them. This also means they can keep raising the prices, and they do, by about 8 to 10% each year, which is more than double compared to the natural and lesser-known brands.

If price is a concern for you, try not to get hooked into buying brand names. Besides, if less of us buy it, maybe they'll lower the prices. Children like what they're used to, so if it's not too late, make the switch. If you don't have any children yet, take it to heart. Don't get them hooked on something you're not willing, or able, to go the distance with.

There is just one more thing to think about when purchasing cereal. It is possible that some of your favorite cereals contain formaldehyde, which is a chemical that is highly toxic to humans. Wheat products treated with formaldehyde do not break down when moistened as quickly as wheat that has not been treated. Many companies will treat the cereal with formaldehyde to keep it crunchy in milk. This is truer for wheat than for corn and some other cereal grains. If you are concerned about this, contact your cereal producer and ask them if they use formaldehyde in production.

Compare and Contrast

Now you've learned the best ways to determine which products are highly processed and which ones are more whole foods oriented. This is the best way to get to know your supermarket and get in the habit of reading labels and making the best choices when you're grocery shopping. Most nutrition and health specialists will agree, reading labels is the most important thing to do at the market.

A good rule to stand by is not purchasing anything that you cannot identify on the label or that has more than five ingredients. This is tough to follow, but it is a nice standard to attempt to maintain. Whatever you do, stay informed and keep reading those labels so you're choosing from a knowledge base and not by auto pilot. I was on auto pilot for a while, thinking I knew what to choose, and I got taken in. Even though they are highly processed, for road trips and easy snacking foods, I was buying some peanut butter pretzels from a name brand I trusted as 'safe' in my opinion. A friend of mine was reading the label and was surprised that they had high fructose corn syrup (HFCS) in them. I stay away from HFCS and don't buy it or let my son ingest it, except with Halloween candy or when it's out of my control, but this shocked me. I had gotten so complacent and, I guess, lazy, that I hadn't bothered reading that label. Needless to say, I don't purchase them anyone and it's something we miss. If I would have followed my own advice from the beginning, we never would have gotten hooked on them and it wouldn't be something we'd be missing now.

What is your shopping style?

Some of us mull about our market and go through it based on our lists. Others go aisle to aisle, pulling whatever looks good off the shelf. Whatever your style of shopping is, get to know your market, so that you know where everything is and don't get trapped by those specials or "sales." Also, try to avoid shopping when you're hungry, that way it will be easier to just say no to all those tasty treats that aren't on your list.

And, please, always bring a list and look it over before you leave the store! Keep a list in your kitchen and as you run out of items write them down, also, check your pantry and fridge for other things you need. Check your list before heading to the store and check it again before getting in line to check out.

Usually the fresher foods are on the perimeter of the store, so try to focus on shopping mainly on the outer ring of the market. All the fresh produce, breads, dairy and meats are the best choices and that's where most of your shopping should be focused.

What's a good way to save time and money and not spend so much on impulse buying?
Shop only once a week and keep a running list.

How do I manage only one trip to the store a week?
Milk delivery!

See if you can get your milk delivered in your neighborhood. Our delivery service also has cheese and meat.

Shopping With Children

If you can avoid shopping with your kids, I highly recommend it; it's probably a good break for us and our kids. When my son was little, we had several markets nearby that had childcare facilities in the store. My son loved it (sometimes) and so did I. Depending on the store, I got one or one-and-a-half hours to shop on my own without little hands grabbing every item they could and placing it in the cart. No whining, no begging: it was great!

If you think the stores with childcare are more expensive, check it out for yourself. Try a store with childcare and one without and compare the price for things you normally purchase. Is there a difference in price? How much is it? How significant is that to you? What are the costs versus benefits to you to pay a little more for a service?

Can you get what you really like at the store that provides childcare?

- ❖ Do they have bulk items?
- ❖ A "Natural Food" section?
- ❖ Certified Organic produce?
- ❖ Uncured, no nitrate/nitrite meats?
- ❖ How far away is it?

What's up with the **"Family Friendly"** checkout stands lately? I went in this aisle thinking *"...alright, no candy and no junk food!"* Oh no, this just meant no magazines. This is the worst checkout stand for me because they've loaded it with all kinds of kid friendly toys and candies right there at a child's eye level, and you name it, my kid wants it!

My son really isn't that bad to shop with, thankfully. However, he's still young and not exposed social pressures yet, plus we don't have a TV, so he's not a victim to what the advertisers want him to want (more about that in the next chapter).

I had a friend who did her shopping at 10 pm while her kids were asleep and home with her husband; she relished her time virtually alone in the store. I've asked my son and he has said he'd rather I do my shopping without him, so for now that's what works best for us. If you and children enjoy shopping together, congratulations, that's terrific!

The Health Food Store

If there is a health food store, what is the food sold in the other stores, non-health food? I'll take the healthy food, thanks! Some supermarkets now have "Natural Food" sections, this makes me wonder too, what is the food in all the other aisles? Non-natural? That's right. I'll stick to natural food as much as I can.

Do you have a Health Food or Natural Food Store near you? How about a Food Cooperative? Have you ever been inside? How often do you shop there?

Step inside a health food store and give it a try. For a dozen years I worked in a Food Cooperative or Health Food Store in just about every city I ever lived in and I think you'll find that the friendly, knowledgeable people who work there really care about your (and their) food supply and the environment.

The health food store is a great place to buy locally grown produce and bulk food items like flour, rice, nuts and herbs and spices. It is much less expensive to buy your food in bulk, because you don't pay for packaging. You also don't have to contribute to all that waste. You can bring in your own containers (be sure to have them weighed by a staff member first), buy containers there, or use the bags provided by the establishment.

The health food store is set up like a supermarket, with similar aisles. Except that the basis of the food inside does not have all the additives and preservatives. Many stores try to purchase local, sustainably grown produce and products. Of course some of the choices are also filled with empty calories, so be sure and read the labels here too, especially on packaged, processed foods.

Why local? Local food is best because it was grown or raised where you live. It comes from the same environment as you, and it is also much fresher and probably less expensive because it didn't have to be shipped, trucked, or trained around the country or world. All those transportation and fuel costs add to the cost of the items you're buying that weren't locally produced.

Sometimes when I'm in a supermarket that sells only conventional foods, it doesn't feel fresh and alive to me, especially the produce aisle. When I go to a natural food store, I can feel that there is more oxygen and more life balance.

Can you notice a difference in your senses when you're in a conventional produce aisle vs. an organic one?

Besides health food stores, many communities have other convenient ways to get fresh local produce, meat and diary products, check your phone book or online for:

- **Community Supported Agriculture (CSA)** –– Farms that deliver (or you pick up) fresh produce weekly or monthly. You pay in advance, which helps support the farm year round. They usually provide recipes and storage tips for the bundles of wonderful fresh fruits and veggies you receive.
- **Milk/Meat Delivery** – The milk man still delivers in my neighborhood. The milk is local, fresh and delicious. Some companies even deliver locally grown meat products, cheese, cookies, coffee, etc...
- **Trader Joe's** – It's not necessarily local, but Trader Joe's has a lot of convenient food items and healthy foods like seeds and nuts. They package most of the food themselves to save money and bring unique items from around the world to your table for reasonable cost. They intentionally buy from vendors that don't

use GMO foods, buy fairly traded products and carry mostly uncured/ nitrate, nitrite free meats, organic, and healthy, whole food products.

Some people think health food stores are more expensive than regular supermarkets. I did a cost comparison on some staple items to see how much of a difference there is in cost. Here's what I discovered:

	Whole Foods – 7/29/09	Safeway – 10/29/09
Milk – ½ gallon, Organic	$3.50	$2.99
Eggs – Cage free	$2.99	$3.99
Flour – All purpose, bleach free	$3.99	$5.49
Bread – 100% whole wheat, organic	$3.29	$2.19
Lettuce – Red leaf, organic	2 for $2.50	$2.49
Total	$15.02	$17.15

For the staple items, the health food store is actually less expensive. For other items, that may not be the case, but overall, there really may not be that much of a difference. Granted I didn't get the chance to shop at these two stores on the same day, week, or even month, so there could be some inflation added into the Safeway total. Check it out for yourself.

Health claims on food packaging

The FDA has regulations about the types of nutrient content and other health claims on food packaging. For instance, claims made about a specific nutrient within the product, can be:

- "No more than two times the type size of the statement of identity" (name of the product). So, you can make a claim that is larger than the actual product name and sometimes it's the claim that sells rather than the actual product itself.

The FDA is currently investigating health claims on food labels because some claims can be misleading. For instance, an item that is almost 50% sugar may have a "Smart Choices" label, whereas, another food package may claim to have a high percent RDI of a certain vitamin, but the product may also contain over 80% of the recommended daily fat intake. The best way to stay healthy and make the best choices is to be aware of the nutrition facts panel and ingredient list. Never mind the health claim, see for yourself and be your own judge.

Some things to consider when making your food purchases:
- ❖ Fat, sugar, and sodium content.
- ❖ Excess packaging: plastics used in packaged processed foods add more waste to our landfills. Much of the shrink-wrapped film covering processed foods is not compostable, recyclable or biodegradable, so it will be with us on the planet for centuries.

Stay supermarket savvy and stay on the healthy highway!

NOTES

Chapter Four

Media Madness

"I find television very educational. Every time someone switches it on I go into another room and read a good book." ~ Groucho Marx

Groucho Marx's sentiment rings true with me. Although I am not against television or mass media (I'm an avid radio listener), I don't own a TV. Television watching was never a habit in the household where I grew up, and in fact, there were restrictions about the shows I was allowed to watch. As I got older, it seemed I only had a television set when I lived in a group house situation, and even then, it was always just *there* to me. In one shared home, I even went into my room and did like Groucho, read a good book, whenever it came on, but it was a small house and that laugh track could really get to me!

I very much appreciated television in the village where I was a Peace Corps Volunteer in West Africa. Sometimes, it was the only thing that brought little bits of familiarity to me. When the TV was brought out around dusk, I would usually be given one of the few lounge chairs underneath the cabana in our little plaza. Only a few times did some bold teenage boy manage to swipe it from me. Oh, how I looked forward to the *Fresh Prince of BelAir!* Now that I'm a single mom, it's not something we choose to spend our monthly budget on. We do check out our fair share of movies at the library, though, and enjoy watching them on our computer.

Whether you're an avid viewer or fly-by watcher, it's worth it to take a close look at what fuels the good ol' *boob tube* as well as other forms of media that we encounter on a daily basis. [1]

---

[1] Much of the following information is adapted from *Media Smart Youth, Eat Think and Be Active!* U.S. Department of Health and Human Services and National Institutes Health, October 2005.

What is the media?

Please, close your eyes and really think about what *media* is.

What does the word *media* mean to you?

You might have come up with something like:
  ❖ Ways of communicating or expressing information or ideas to people.
  ❖ Examples of media: newspapers, radio, books, letters, recorded music, the Internet, television, and telephone calls.

How many different types of media can you name?

Did you think of all these, or more?

• Newspaper • TV • Radio • Books • Magazines • Music • Internet • Billboards • Movies • Videos • Visual Art (paintings, photos, sculptures, etc.) • Theater • Dance • Performance Art • IPod/Zune • TIVO	• Video games • Comic books/ graphic novels • Advertisements/ commercials • Infomercials • Public Service Announcements • Signs on the outside or inside of buses or at bus stops/ transit stops • Radio contests • Art contests • Signs on the sides of trucks and vans • Food or drink packages (for example, cereal boxes) • Mail/ e-mail/instant messaging • Telephone/text messages • Flyers/ brochures

Which types of media are you most exposed to? Depending on the number of hours you spend watching television, advertisements and commercials could be in the top three media that you are exposed to.

Seriously ask yourself the question, *"What is the purpose of media? Why do we have media?"*

Media delivers a product and each product serves a purpose or reason for having been created.

All media products have a purpose

There are **three main purposes** of media. They are:

1) To **entertain** (for example, comic books or movies)
2) To **inform** (for example, TV or radio news)
3) To **persuade** (for example, magazine or TV advertisements)

Some types of media may have more than one purpose, and some, like television, serves all of the three of the main purposes and then some.

Why is it helpful to know the different kinds of media?

❖ Knowing the purpose helps us to be more aware of how media is used and how media may affect us.
❖ Knowing the purpose helps us to think critically about what we see and hear in the media.

Media and health

Media can influence people's attitudes and decisions about many things, especially nutrition, physical activity, and body image.

How much time each day do you spend, on average, using media?

Using media includes behaviors such as playing video games, listening to music, reading, using the computer, and watching TV, videotapes, or DVD's. Even reading this book!

How much time do you think the average young person spends using media?

According to a 2004 study titled *Kids & Media in America,* young people ages 11 to 14 spend an average of **6 hours and 45 minutes** a day using media. This is more than they spend doing anything else except sleeping!

What are your thoughts about this amount of time?

Are you close to any young people? If so,
- What kind of media do you think they're most exposed to?
- How much time do they spend with each form of media?

My hunch is that the majority of that media time is "screen time". Instead of sitting in front of a video screen or even reading magazines, or non-school related media, what else could young people (or you, if you also put in too much screen time) do with all that extra time?

Instead of screen time try:
- Going for a walk with friend(s)
- Doing homework, or work on an art project, like drawing or poetry
- Playing sports or games with friends or family
- Going roller/in-line skating
- Riding a bike
- Flying a kite
- Talking with someone (not texting!)
- Taking care of errands
- Doing household chores (like vacuum, sweep, wash windows, etc.)
- Gardening
- Cooking -- share food or recipes with neighbors
- Hula Hoop – learn how to make your own in the next chapter.

Hundreds of studies on the effects of TV violence on children and teenagers have found that children may:
<ul><li>Become "immune" or numb to the horror of violence</li><li>Gradually accept violence as a way to solve problems</li><li>Imitate the violence they observe on television; and</li><li>Identify with certain characters, victims and/or victimizers</li></ul>

Violence on TV has increased significantly in the last 30 years; violence in schools has increased in the exact same amount: 300 percent! Violence is not healthy for anyone.

So, what's the health connection?

❖ Media is everywhere and can have a powerful effect on our attitudes, behaviors and health. Think about the purpose of all the magazines at the check-out stand in the grocery stores, or even the video-streamed ads at supermarkets and gas pumps.

❖ The majority of food being advertised is high in fat and added sugar and do not have much nutritional value. *What is the purpose of those ads?* To sell as much **high-profit** product as possible.

❖ Many people like to snack while they use a type of media and do not realize how much they are eating. They often choose high-fat, high-added sugar foods that taste good and fill them up, but may not have much nutritional value. Research shows people tend to eat more when they're distracted, and this can add up to eating 21% more chips while watching TV than you would by snacking without distraction.

❖ Foods are often made to look very tempting. TV ads link eating with "fun" and "excitement", which can override eating to satisfy hunger. People are more likely to overeat if they lose track of whether or not they are hungry. So ask yourself, *"Am I hungry?"* before you take a bite of food.

❖ Attractive role models can inspire us to take care of our bodies by eating smart and being active. But some body sizes and shapes portrayed are unrealistic and have little to do with being healthy.

❖ We're kept busy but not necessarily active. People often choose to use media instead of being physically active.

❖ Sports are often portrayed as fun and exciting. Although that portrayal encourages an interest in sports, some people watch sports on TV instead of personally being active.

Why do most people spend more time using media than they do being physically active?

Whose point of view?

As a media user, it's a good idea to acknowledge where the point of view is coming from. *What does point of view mean to you?*

It might mean:

❖ The way that someone looks at or interprets a specific situation or issue, or someone's perspective on an issue.
❖ The position from which something is considered.

Why should you consider the point of view presented in media?
- The same topic or issue often can be perceived from many different perspectives.
- Knowing the point of view that is presented in media can help you understand the information you see and hear.
- People may form different opinions about a topic, depending on the points of view they are exposed to in the media.

What's in the packaging?

Much of media is wrapped up in a shiny package called advertising!

Well, what is an advertisement?

❖ An advertisement is an announcement designed to attract people's attention.
❖ It is a specific kind of media with the main purpose being to persuade people to buy or support something – a product, service, or belief.

When you think of advertisements, what is the first thing that comes to your mind?

What types of advertising do you encounter on a typical day?

How often do you observe any of these?

- ✓ Billboards
- ✓ Cups and mugs
- ✓ Food and drink packages
- ✓ Infomercials (30-minute programs that promote a product or service)
- ✓ Internet pop-up ads
- ✓ Logos
- ✓ Magazine ads
- ✓ Mail
- ✓ Newspaper ads
- ✓ Previews before movies and videos (rentals or in the theater)
- ✓ Promotional activities in schools
- ✓ Public service announcements (print, TV, or radio)
- ✓ Radio commercials
- ✓ School cafeterias/ vending machines
- ✓ Shopping bags
- ✓ Shopping malls
- ✓ Signs in sports stadiums
- ✓ Signs on the outsides and/or insides of buses
- ✓ Signs on the sides of trucks and vans
- ✓ Telemarketing
- ✓ TV commercials

Some things to consider about advertising:

- ❖ It is all around us, in many parts of our lives
- ❖ There are many different ways to advertise.
- ❖ Advertising appears in places we may not immediately think of, such as on cereal boxes or other product packages. Some supermarket check-out stands and gas stations have mini TVs that display shows as well as advertisements.

Some advertising is blatant or obvious, but some advertising is not so obvious and is subtle, which is not direct, but something that can be hard to detect or analyze.

Two forms of subtle advertising:
Logos
Product Placement

What is a logo?

- ❖ A logo is a symbol that stands for a company and its beliefs.
- ❖ A logo aims to make you recognize, be familiar with, and like a product.

Are you wearing any items with a logo(s) on them? How many?

To some people, logos are very important. *Why do you think many people feel it is important to wear clothes with particular logos on them?*

- ❖ They want to be associated with products or companies or teams that they think are cool or represent a certain lifestyle, faith, or attitude.
- ❖ They see people they like wearing them, such as actors, musicians, athletes, or friends.
- ❖ Many of these products are heavily advertised: seeing them often makes people want to have them.

What is product placement?

❖ Companies pay to have their products placed in specific films and TV shows.

❖ Companies also pay to have their products appear in video games, books, websites, music lyrics, and comic books.

Why is product placement such an effective form of advertising?

❖ From the audience's point of view, it looks like the product just "happens" to be there, but it is put there for the purpose of marketing it to the show's audience.

❖ We want to be like the actors and celebrities in TV shows and movies who use those products.

❖ Seeing a particular product in places that we go or watch – even in TV shows and the movies – makes it seem as though it's everywhere.

❖ Companies want you to see their products because, when you think about needing a certain item, you are more likely to think of using their brand.

> *Have you noticed how much product placement is on the rise?* Not only in TV shows and movies, but children's books, even textbooks! Due to budget cuts, many schools receive corporate sponsorship today, so they have no choice but to open their doors to advertising.

Branding is another type of advertising that is focused on youth. If a company can get a young person so used to seeing their product that it is "branded" in their brain, they will have a customer for life.

> **The younger a child is when a product or company is *branded* into their brain, the more loyal that child will be to that brand for the rest of his or her life!**

What do you think the effect of all these forms of advertising has on our lives and that of our children?

- ❖ Advertising makes us want the products we see promoted.
- ❖ We associate certain products with specific ways of being, such as being beautiful, happy, carefree, popular, rich, or smart.
- ❖ We associate certain actors or music with specific products.
- ❖ Advertising affects our emotions by portraying the way we want to feel about ourselves.

Advertising targeted to children in the U.S. is estimated at more than $16.8 billion annually, more than twice what it was in 1992.

How many ads do you think you see and hear every year? Youth see and hear an average of 40,000 advertisements a year. Most of these advertisements are for food – mainly candy, cereal, and fast food.

What does all this food advertising do for our children?

- ❖ It gives children a lot of attention, but it is not necessarily good for them.
- ❖ Food advertisements promote processed foods and foods that are high in fat and added sugar more than they promote fruits and vegetables, whole grains, and foods that are low in fat and added sugar.
- ❖ It can be hard to choose healthy foods when there is so much focus on foods that are high in fat and added sugar in the media. With all that attention, the less healthy foods can be hard to resist.

What about school lunches? If you are unhappy with the food being sold or advertised at your school, get involved! Parents and teachers must request healthy choices in schools. Let the school board know you would like to see improvements in the school lunch program. Children go to school to learn, some parents don't have a lot of education, so they learn from their children.

Schools should role model healthy lifestyles by not allowing unhealthy foods on campus!

Yes, I'm sorry to say I'm talking about those birthday cupcakes. Let those treats be special ones shared at home. Children go to school to learn and they should learn that sugar is not the best fuel for our bodies. What else could we do to celebrate our children's birthday without having to bring sugary sweets to school? I realize this is a tough one to tackle and I don't have the answer but maybe it is something we should be mindful of...

Five media questions

There are five basic questions to ask in order to make an informed decision about what you're being exposed to in the media:

1. Who is the sponsor or author?
   ❖ The media product shows the name of a company, group, or person it is from, or it says "sponsored by" or "brought to you by."
   ❖ The media product shows a logo that you identify with a specific company, group, or person.
   ❖ The media product uses colors or music that you associate with a particular company, group, or person.

   Why is it important to know the sponsor?
   • To help you understand the point of view of the message.
   • To help you understand why you are being asked to take a certain action.
   • To help form an opinion about the message.

It's also wise to know the sponsor of particular studies, politicians, or even professional organizations – that way you can understand why they make the decisions they do and what the real purpose (or agenda) is.

2. Who is the audience they're targeting?
- ❖ Who is the product geared towards? In other words, who is meant to see, hear, or use the product?

3. What is the purpose of the media product?
- ❖ To entertain
- ❖ To inform
- ❖ To persuade/ influence
- ❖ To sell something, i.e. make money

Keep the purpose in mind, as it is often the agenda behind the pretty package. Sometimes the agenda, or purpose is hidden, and you have to work hard to uncover it.

4. What information is being given?
- ❖ The message, point, or opinion being expressed.
- ❖ What are people being told? Ever think about what information is being left out?

5. What techniques are being used to attract attention?
- ❖ Sound, color, humor, celebrities, fear, etc…
- ❖ Different techniques work for different audiences.

Let's look at this book as an example of a type of media:
1. **Who is the author?** Me, I'm a nutrition, health and wellness consultant, Returned Peace Corps Volunteer, and low income and underserved population advocate.
2. **Who is the audience trying to be reached?** People who want to make the best choices for their bodies, but might not know where to start, or who may need a gentle reminder of all the good reasons to make the best choices they can, most of the time.
3. **What is the purpose of the media product?** To inform, and, let's face it, persuade you to look at your lifestyle and possibly make some changes.
4. **What information is being given?** Nutrition information to help people better understand their bodies.
5. **What techniques are being used to attract attention?** Possible mass marketing.

Bringing it home

Hopefully, this chapter helped you to be more informed about media, how much of it we're exposed to, and what a big influence it has on our daily lives and the choices we make. Before you get drawn into a particular product or cause, stop and think about the five media questions and decide for yourself what to do. Your best interests may not be the purpose of that media you're watching.

In 1997, $7 billion was spent on food advertising, the majority of which most of us would consider junk food. That same year, the USDA spent only $333 *million* on nutrition related education: that's only 5% of the junk food industry's spending.

Today, 13 years later, the food advertising budget has doubled, but the USDA nutrition education budget hasn't made any headway. The junk food industry spends 200% more on advertising than the health food industry. Those odds are hard to beat for anyone wanting to make the right food choices. It's a long road, but with the knowledge and know-how, you can help yourself, friends and loved ones read through the media messages and make the best choices when making food purchases.

There are many reasons food is so highly advertised and marketed, but mainly it is because we all need to eat, so it's what is considered a "repeat" purchase item, meaning we always go back for more. The food items that are most highly advertised are the ones that make the largest profit. That's why "junk food" is so heavily advertised. It's cheap to make and gains the highest profit margin!

Don't get caught up in the media madness. Take control of your choices and buy what's best for you, not what the advertisers want to sell you!

NOTES

Chapter Five

Movement Matters

After dinner sit a while, and after supper walk a mile ~ English Saying

---

The end all, be all, in cruising *your* vehicle through *your* Sun, Moon, or Sky, is movement!

Imagine it!

Close your eyes and picture your vehicle cruising around in your frame!

Why Movement Matters So Much

All machines would prefer to do the job for which they were created, rather than rust in the shed. Your body is no different. It wants to move and groove as much as it can. So get up and get going! Whatever it is your body likes to and can do, do it! And don't forget to breathe while you're at...I'm talking big huge, deep, meaningful, powerful, loud, intoxicating breaths!

Even if you don't have the time, money, or desire for a fitness club, get out there and move that thing. Whatever it is you do in a day, do it more, shake in your seat if you have to, just move!!! Should I get into the studies about how movement is the key to health and longevity? There is plenty of evidence on the benefits of exercise and chances are we've all heard it over and over again. Exercise releases hormones called endorphins that are feel good receptors in our brains, so it can help relieve stress, combat anxiety and depression. Without exercise, the chances of reversing many of the obesity-related diseases we've discussed, including Type 2 Diabetes are minimal. You can't just eat right to get healthy and you can't just exercise to get healthy. It's a two-way street: you have to incorporate both. Research even shows that regular exercise; four to six days a week reduces the length and intensity of menopause symptoms.

C'mon, it's only 30 to 60 minutes a day. Is that really too much for your body to ask from you? The body was designed to hunt and gather, as in run and stretch, not eat and sit around! Our bodies were made to move, not lay on a couch! So if you want to "veg out" in front of the television, please shake your saddle a little! And eat your veggies while you're doing it, not those too fatty, too salty *poisons* they sell at the "super" market.

If you have to break it up into 10 minutes at a time, that's fine, just do it, and add it up! It doesn't matter how you fit movement into your daily routine, your body will thank you and repay you in kind. Skip on your way to the mail box, or park just those extra hundred feet further away or how about taking the bus instead of your car one day a week?

You can take a walk, skip, or dance: it's free and it makes you feel better! If you live in a city where it is unsafe to walk outside, you'll just have to dance around your living room, so put on your tunes and bounce! You can even stand in your living room and *hula hoop* (learn how to make one easily and cheaply in this chapter). A current golden rule is to achieve 10,000 steps a day; many people have pedometers that measure every step they take to help them with this goal. Ten thousand is quite a few steps, but should be fairly easy to manage if you do your daily 30 to 60 minutes of exercise. If you can't get a pedometer, no problem, just make sure you move your body the required 30 to 60 minutes most days of the week.

One thing that may be good to know is that will power is actually a muscle in our brain! This is great because like any muscle, the willpower muscle can be trained and toned and with practice, it gets stronger. So, getting out there and getting physical today could help you do the same tomorrow. This same will power helps you to refrain from taking that second helping of mashed potatoes; saying no to something at lunch, could help you say no at dinner, too!

Let's get physical

Below is a list of exercises that just about anyone can do. I try to give examples and elaborate as much as possible on the movements and postures. However, if you need more information on any of these topics, it's all available on the web, which you can access at any library if you don't own a computer.

I make the following movement recommendations to everyone, but I am not a physical therapist, and can't know your particular situation. If you have any medical conditions that inhibit you from physical activity, please try the ones that seem reasonable for you. Or, give your doctor a copy of this book and ask him what you can do it get more movement into your lifestyle.

Whatever it is you do for a living, whether you're in grade school, or grad school, whether you're a teenager or grandmother, you can probably do many of these exercises on your living room floor, at your desk at work, or in your dorm room.

Stretches *

What do animals and babies have in common? Stretching! Have you ever noticed that babies stretch their little bodies a lot, especially after waking up? What about your favorite pet, do you notice how they stretch whenever they get up from lounging? What happened to us? Most people over the age of three that I know do not stretch very often. Stretching's a good habit to get into, it loosens your muscles and joints and helps relieve stress and tension. I live near Seattle, where Ichiro Suzuki plays for the Mariner's baseball team. Have you ever watched how much he stretches and moves to keep limber? He's an amazing athlete and a good example of how to keep your body pliable. Go ahead, stretch!

The following is a list of stretches to do any time. Make your routine and do them whenever you feel tight, wake up in the morning, get off the couch, or step away from your computer. They are also great stretches to do before and after your fitness routine. Stretching helps counteract any tightness you may feel from your exercises.

The Technique
- Relax into the stretch, especially your shoulders.
- Take deep breaths as you start each stretch. Inhale through your nose and slowly exhale through your mouth.
- Don't bounce or force the stretch
- Hold the stretch for 5 to 10 seconds, ease off, and then relax into the stretch again for another 5 to 10 seconds.

Arm stretch Standing tall, lift your arms straight above your head and bend at your elbow and try to hold your hands together.

Calf stretch Stand slightly facing a wall. Place hands flat on wall and lean in on your forearms, resting your head on your hands. Bend right leg out in front of you with toe and knee against the wall. Straighten your left leg out behind you. Keep your lower back flat, both heels on the floor, toes straight ahead and press your back heel into the floor, holding the stretch. Switch legs.

Chest stretch While sitting or standing, reach behind you and grasp your hands together. Pull up slightly and hold for 4 counts. Do this 10 times.

Hamstring stretch Sitting with right leg straight, bend left leg with sole against the inside of right thigh. Lean down over right leg and reach out, grab your ankle (if you can), slowly bending forward from your hips towards your ankle, keeping your right leg straight and your head help up. Alternate legs.

Lower Leg Lie on back. Raise one knee to your chest, and grasping the knee; pull it in towards your chest. Hold the stretch until you can feel it. Relax and repeat 5 times. Do the same stretch with the opposite leg, then both legs together.

Quadriceps stretch Stand tall with shoulders over hips, bend right knee and grasp ankle with left hand. Pull ankle toward your bottom until you feel the stretch. Switch legs. You may need to balance yourself by resting your hand on a wall or chair back.

* Injuries can occur during stretching because of poor technique. Please be gentle, don't force a stretch, relax and breathe, completely, deeply and peacefully!!

The Movements

For ease and convenience, the movements are alphabetized. Try them all if you can, or pick and choose what's right for you. These are simple exercises to do while watching TV, sitting at your desk, or on your living room floor. If you're already active and you stay physically fit, good for you!!!! Keep it up, try something new, and always remember to breathe deeply and often.

Backwards push ups – Sit on floor, put arms out behind you, hands flat on floor with fingers facing towards your bottom. Bend knees so feet are flat on the floor and lift your arms until your bottom is a couple of inches off the floor. Do not use your legs for this, use only your arms. Do 12 counts.

Hula hoop You can make your own high quality hula hoop at minimal cost! The hula hoops sold at local dollar stores are usually poor quality and don't function properly because they're too light, the heavier the hula hoop, the easier it is to use! It's simple to make your own; just go to your neighborhood hardware store and buy ¾ inch PVC piping, some connectors (ask for help if you need it) and colorful duct or electrical tape. Cut (or saw) the piping into 5 to 6 foot lengths (or ask the associate at the hardware store to cut it for you), heat the ends in hot water and add the connectors. Wrap your hula hoop with your tape, 2 or 3 colors look great! Using this is excellent exercise you can do just about anywhere as long you have enough room.

Leg lifts While seated, bend knees so feet touch the ground, then lift your legs straight out and hold for 4 counts. Do this 10 times.

Lunch fitness routine – If you're an office worker and you have access to a room you can reserve, plan a *"movement matters lunchercise"* with your coworkers and do some of the movements in this chapter, or ask a professional to come in and offer a yoga class or something you'll all enjoy. Or map out a 30-minute route you can walk together or alone.

Lunges With hands on hips, stand with feet a shoulder width apart, step right foot out in front of you as if you're taking a step. Now, bend down until left knee almost touches the floor, hold for 3 counts. Lift yourself back up, return to standing, do the same with left foot out in front. Do this 10 times.

Sit ups/ crunches Lay on the floor; bend knees so feet are flat on the floor. Hold hands behind your head with elbows in line with your shoulders. Lift your head and shoulders, tucking tummy inwards and holding tight. Do 20 counts.

Sit up variation A great variation on the sit-up: lay on the floor, feet stretched straight out, hands under your hips. Bending legs at hips lift them straight up, then lower legs until they barely hit the floor. Relax, do 20 counts.

Tai Chi This is a mild Chinese form of martial art that is invigorating, yet relaxing, and most anyone of any fitness level can do it. It's similar to yoga, in that once you learn the moves you are empowered with an easy, free form of exercise anywhere you go. Look for Tai Chi classes in local gyms, books, park districts, or on YouTube.

Waist crunches While seated or standing, twist at your waist for 2 counts, and then switch sides. Do this 20 times on each side.

Walk Plan a 30 to 60 minute walk around your neighborhood if you can: your body won't mind if you walk even longer. Living in the Northwest, we have a lot of ferry commuters, our local cooperative hospital mapped out a walk routine for people to follow while on their commute, instead of sitting in their cars. What a great idea! Get up every so often and walk around your office building: your co-workers should understand and will probably respect you for it.

Yoga I cannot do justice to all the poses and postures involved in the different practices of the art of yoga and won't attempt to, as I'm not a yoga instructor. Yoga is great strengthening exercise and most poses can be modified to adjust to almost any ability level. Many community centers and city/county park districts offer low-cost classes these days; and you can check out a book or video from the library. My first yoga book was *Elements of Yoga* by Godfrey Devereux. Once you learn the poses, you'll have them to help keep you fit for the rest of your life.

Calorie Burner Guide

Many of our daily activities burn quite a few calories... The following chart estimates calories burned per activity per minute. The actual number of calories you burn will vary with your body weight, as indicated by the chart, the more you weigh, the more calories you burn.

Activity	Weight: 105 - 115	Weight: 127 - 137	Weight: 160 - 170	Weight: 180 - 200
Basketball	9.8	11.2	13.2	14.5
Bicycling - Stationary	5.5	6.3	7.8	8.3
Bicycling - Stationary 20 mph	11.7	13.3	15.6	17.8
Bicycling - 10 mph	5.5	6.3	7.8	14.5
Dancing	3.3	3.8	4.4	4.9
Golfing	3.3	3.8	4.4	4.9
Hiking	5.9	6.7	7.9	8.8
Jogging - 5 mph	8.6	9.2	11.5	12.7
Lawn Mowing	3.5	4.0	4.8	5.2
Running - 8 mph	10.4	11.9	14.2	17.3
Skating	8.1	9.3	10.9	12
Skiing - down hill	7.8	10.4	12.3	13.3
Skiing - cross country	13.1	15	17.8	19.4
Snow shoveling	7.9	9.1	10.8	12.5
Stair Climbing	5.9	6.7	7.9	8.8
Swimming	3.9	4.5	5.3	6.8
Tennis (singles)	7.8	8.9	10.5	11.6
Volleyball	7.8	8.9	10.5	11.6
Walking, 2 mph	2.4	2.8	3.3	3.6
Walking 4 mph	4.5	5.2	6.1	6.8

Do you wonder why watching TV is not on the list? Watching TV is not exercise. When I was in college, I remember reading a research study that indicated a person burns more calories staring at a blank wall than watching TV. The theory behind it is that TV watching is a very passive activity, whereas staring at a blank wall requires more energy, because your eyes are probably moving more rapidly and you may even make more body movements, like fidgeting. When you watch TV, you usually sit there and don't move a muscle for a very long time.

Pre and Post Workout Snacks

Before and after your workout you may want to eat foods to replace the nutrients used up during your workout. The amount of fuel you need to replace depends on the amount of exercise you perform. If you're an endurance athlete, like a marathon runner or cyclist, your body has higher recovery needs.

Pre Workout Snacks:
About an hour before you workout, eat a combination of carbohydrates and proteins. The carbs help maintain energy during your workout and prevent depletion of glycogen stores. The amino acids in protein are available and used by muscles when consumed before your workout and help in post workout recovery.

Here are some examples:
- ½ bagel with 1 tbsp of peanut/almond butter
- ½ cup granola with ½ cup yogurt
- multi grain cereal with berries and 1 cup of (non-fat) milk
- dried fruit and nuts/ seeds (apricots with almonds)
- banana and yogurt
- cottage cheese with honey

Post workout Snacks:
After the workout, you have used up some of your glycogen, so you need to replace it with more carbohydrates. You also need protein to help rebuild muscle tissues. A good balance of carbs and proteins is the best snack for post workout recovery. If you don't replace the protein used up in your workout, your body is likely to get it from your muscles, this would defeat the whole purpose of your workout.

A well balanced meal is ideal:
- Smoothie with yogurt and banana, other fruit and whey protein
- Turkey sandwich on whole wheat bread with lettuce, tomato, cucumber, a tad of mayo and fruit on the side
- Chicken wrapped in tortilla with veggies and a glass of (nonfat) milk
- Chicken and vegetable stir fry with brown rice

If you don't have time, etc. for a meal post workout, have a snack such as:
- Sliced turkey, cheese, fruit
- Tuna with whole wheat crackers
- Banana and (nonfat) milk

*Remember starving yourself before a workout won't cause you to loose more weight or burn more calories, the opposite will happen because you won't be able to work out as hard and will burn less efficiently.

Go on, get out there, and move that wonderful machine of yours! Breathe, drink your water and enjoy!

NOTES

Chapter Six

The Road Map

Keeping your body healthy is an expression of gratitude to the whole cosmos - the trees, the clouds, every thing ~ Thich Nhat Hanh

Think of this chapter as a GPS for how to effectively and efficiently cruise through life on the highway to health. There is a fork in the road, the choice is yours: take the healthy route.

If you're serious about cruising down the highway to health, go out and buy a journal, or make your own out of plain paper or a notebook. Whatever you do, just start making lists and journaling. Here's a fact about dieters: studies show that dieters who keep a daily journal of all the food they eat are twice as successful at eating right as those who don't. Two times as successful! That's huge. 200%! This doesn't have to relate to just people who want to lose weight, we are all dieters in that we all have to eat every day. A diet simply refers to an eating plan. So whether your goal is weight loss or weight gain, or to be healthier and make better choices, journaling will help you on your path. All you have to do is write down everything you eat to have double the outcome. Terrific!

The Positive Approach

A good way to set out on the *highway to health* is to focus on what's going well with your body and health. Don't focus on what's going wrong. Whatever we focus on is what we attract. So, if we focus on the negative, that's the thing that will continue. Focus on the positive!

If you know what's going well and focus on doing the right thing, you can improve on that and keep it up. Soon you'll be making all the healthy choices (well, maybe not **all**, none of us are perfect and there sure are a lot of choices out there).

Start with a list of your current behaviors and move on from there to keep making improvements in your day-to-day life.

Current Behaviors:
What are the things you currently do that are in line with a healthy lifestyle?

Highway to Health:
What would you like to add to the list above?

Keep doing the things that are on your list of current behaviors and add the things in your highway to health list. If you keep this lifestyle up, pretty soon most of your behaviors will be healthy ones. Just keep adding new things to your healthy highway list and you'll be traveling in the fast lane and feeling free.

Of course, there will always be setbacks and cravings, and as long as most of your choices are the best ones, you'll be doing great! Don't beat yourself up about making wrong turns and getting lost. If you steer yourself off track, remember to steer yourself back on, the same day if possible. Waiting until tomorrow or next Monday to get back on track may let guilt creep onto the scene and that can lead you down a vicious, unproductive path. Find your way back on the healthy highway as soon as possible, and as long as you keep your eye on the road ahead you'll be doing better and feeling happier.

We are living in the time of the information age: 2010 is here. There is a world of information at our fingertips on this *information highway*. Harness that knowledge, make the wisest choices, and ride the highway to health!

Emotional Intelligence

We are inundated with information that is loaded with stimulus and advertising. Use your emotional intelligence (EQ) and make healthy choices.

When you pause before making a decision, you get a second chance, another choice to do the right thing. Doing the right thing feels good and your body feels good when it's fed healthy food.

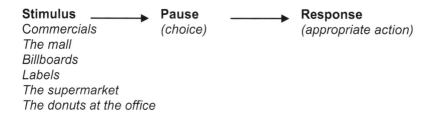

Stimulus ⟶ Pause ⟶ Response
Commercials *(choice)* *(appropriate action)*
The mall
Billboards
Labels
The supermarket
The donuts at the office

We need to slow down and pause before we respond to the stimulus we're surrounded by. As noted motivational speaker Stephen Covey explains, when we receive stimulus, such as a brownie, we should pause for a flash and think about that brownie and what it does to our bodily systems. In that pause we have space, and within that space lays our choice. That choice makes us feel good, which correlates to happiness.

Choice is something we all have to deal with every day; some of us have more choice than others. Some of us make better choices with the resources and information we have. I have weaknesses just as much as the next person and I know when I'm making a bad choice. I don't hate myself for it; I just decide whether I'm going to continue to let myself make unwise choices or do better next time. Also, just because I chose to eat a few donuts this morning doesn't mean I have to stay out of control the rest of the day, or week. I just jump right back on the highway and continue my journey, because *a little flat tire ain't gonna stop me from getting to my destination.*

- **Natural Intelligence**

Some may also want to draw upon our *Natural Intelligence*. Natural intelligence is what tells us something is right and true for us. We have lost touch with our natural intelligence, but with practice you can get it back. I like to consider my body as it would be 1,000 years ago, what would have been my body's needs for fuel then? Realistically, our bodies have not changed their requirements throughout millennium, what changed is our food supply and the way we get our food. Pause before making a choice and think: "is this something my body would have ever come across a thousand or even a hundred years ago?" If not, then it is not the natural intelligence choice and maybe something you don't want to put into your precious system too often.

Take jelly beans for instance, they are made of basically corn syrup and food coloring, I don't know anyone who has ever made their own jelly beans at home. I don't have anything against jelly beans and once a year, I like to indulge in eating a few, just a few. However, they are a good example and there are many ways of looking at them, and if you look at them through your natural intelligence you'll see that there is nothing natural about a jelly bean. If you were a body walking around with only natural food choices, you would never stumble upon jelly beans, so choosing a jelly bean is not a natural choice.

If you look around the lunchroom, or in your kitchen, hopefully you will find natural choices, like raw almonds, or fruit. Those are choices from nature's intelligence. In order to make the most of this option, you'll have to make sure your office, kitchen and meeting rooms are well stocked with natural intelligence selections. For the most part, I'll choose nature's intelligence over *chemical intelligence.* In my opinion, chemical intelligence would be jelly beans, or things food chemists came up with. Take the quote at the beginning of Chapter 2; trusting cows more than chemists is another way of saying you trust natural intelligence more than chemical intelligence, at least when it comes to food. Of course, chemists have made great advances in our food supply with things like pasteurization and the like; however nature still wins in my book.

> **There is power in knowing you have the choice. Knowledge is power! Now that you have the knowledge, do you have the motivation to harness that power?**

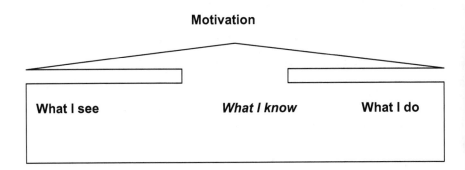

The Road Ahead

A good idea to get started on your road ahead is to find out how many calories your particular machine requires to run itself on a daily basis (base caloric intake). The United States Department of Agriculture (USDA) has developed a website solely for the purpose of helping you determine your daily caloric intake and it even has meal plans and ideas of how to go about it. Log onto **www.mypyramid.gov** go to the left column, click on Mypyramid Plan and enter your personal information. It'll tell you how much you should eat and give you the appropriate macronutrient ratios you need to maintain your current weight. It'll also tell you if you should lose or gain weight and will give you some suggestions on how to do that.

A study published in Science Magazine revealed that 90% of adults can prevent gaining weight by simply increasing their physical activity level by 2,000 steps and eating 100 fewer calories a day. That should be fairly easy to accomplish and doesn't require 'dieting' at all. You may not lose weight that way, but you certainly won't gain any, and that's a good start.

Weight Loss

If you want to lose some weight, make sure you're eating enough. That's right, eating enough! I've found in my practice that many of my clients simply aren't eating enough… they aren't eating breakfast, they aren't eating snacks, they aren't eating enough vegetables, enough fiber, you name it, they aren't eating enough. They may have been eating so little for so long that their metabolism has slowed down significantly, so what they do eat gets stored as fat because their poor body is worried about when it's going to get fed again.

If you are on, or are planning to go on a weight loss diet, you need to find out what your base caloric intake is so that you know where you need to be in order to maintain a healthy weight. If you eat too much below that amount for too long, you'll reach that *dieter's plateau* and won't lose anymore. If you go above that without burning it, you'll gain more.

- To lose weight, eat a few hundred calories (some may want to restrict by 500) fewer than your base caloric intake for a month, then go to your base level for a month in order to boost your metabolism and continue on like this until you reach your ideal weight.
- When you reach your ideal weight, stick to your base caloric intake level while continuing to exercise and you should be able to keep your weight stable. It's kind of like a dance, restrict your calories then increase, restrict, increase, etc. This way you don't 'starve' yourself for too long and lower your metabolism for too long, by eating more, you actually increase your metabolism.
- Realize you didn't gain your weight overnight and you're not going to lose it overnight either, so don't stress, don't kick yourself and don't hurt yourself by restricting calories for too long. If you have any questions or concerns, consult your doctor, or see a nutrition specialist.

To maintain your current weight, find out your maintenance calories (base caloric intake). Then strive to not go over that and be sure to get in 30 minutes of physical activity. Remember: 90% of adults can prevent gaining weight by taking 2,000 extra steps a day and eating only 100 fewer calories!

Snacks

Have you heard the term *you have to eat to lose?* It doesn't initially make sense, does it? Well, what it means is that you have to eat more often and more of the good stuff. Eating snacks is a great plan for nearly anyone. As we've learned, the whole digestive process takes about six hours, but within that time your body is ready for more fuel. In order to keep your metabolism pumping hard, feed it a little something every three or four hours. Some frame types can get by without snacks, although in my practice I've found that most people do better when they include a mid-morning and/or mid-afternoon snack. Because I'm so small and wiry, I have to eat every couple of hours or I don't feel right.

I have numerous quotes from clients who are amazed at how much weight they have lost by eating more. Eating more doesn't necessarily mean more food, remember, not more than your base caloric intake, or what you burn in a day. What it means is to eat healthy and nutritious foods more often. Large people who have had a lot to lose have told me they can't believe how much they're eating, yet how much they lose by following basically everything in this book. Much of this is because my clients are now eating snacks and being mindful of their bodies' needs. My clients' chronic problems with heartburn disappear, they go off blood pressure medication and squelch pre-diabetes. They feel well fed and full.

My favorite snack has always been a couple small pieces of dried fruit and a few nuts or seeds; they are sweet and satisfying and pack a lot of nutrition to fuel you through to the next meal. I enjoy most dried fruits, and while papaya is my favorite, I also like dates, figs, and apricots. Beware; some dried fruits have added sugar, so read those labels. For nuts I usually stick to raw almonds (their health benefits are numerous) and pumpkin or sunflower seeds. If I'm a little hungrier, I might also munch on some ginger snaps (I like gluten free ones) or granola and yogurt with my dried fruit, seeds and nuts. If I'm just craving chocolate or something extra sweet, I might grab a couple chocolate chips. You'll be pleasantly surprised: just a few will do.

Some research suggests that by actually taking smaller bites of food our bodies still get the sensations of the meal (taste, texture, aroma – the good stuff to get digestion going), but we consume less food. This translates into using smaller plates so you take smaller portions, but also, use smaller utensils, like a teaspoon for ice cream instead of a soup spoon. That way you'll still get the sensory exposure without all the excess calories, fat, sugar, etc.

The Golden Rule for Eaters:

- **Eat upon rising in the morning** (within an hour of waking up), this gets your metabolism fire burning good and strong throughout the day.
- **Continue to eat a little bit every few hours.** Some frames can deal with only "three square meals" and no snacks, while many people do better on more frequent, smaller meals. Test drive your rig and see how it runs best.
- **Don't eat anything for two or three hours before going to bed.** This isn't so much because you'll gain weight overnight, but to slow down your metabolism while you're resting, making sure you're good and hungry when you get up in the morning, so you feed your body and keep it running throughout the day.
- **Don't overdo it and put more fuel in your tank than what it'll hold** (don't go over your base caloric intake without working it off) or it will spill over and onto your thighs, your hips, your tush, your neck, your arms, or your stomach. That may not be so bad to you, but when it spills over into your arteries and organs, such as your liver, you're headed for the highway to the hospital.

The "Diet"

I teach my clients and classes about healthy choices and encourage them to make small, slow lifestyle changes. I encourage them to think in terms of weekly changes, it isn't about making giant steps everyday. To get them on their way prior to having a chance to really get a meal plan in place, I give them a copy of the chart below (as well as a list of foods for their frame type, see Chapter 1). For each meal listed, choose an item from the food group indicated by the corresponding letter. Remember not to go over your recommended calorie intake or the excess, if not burned off, will be stored somewhere in your body.

This diet plan is just an idea and may not be right for everyone, but a lot of people need something to follow to help them make choices for each meal and snack of the day. It is not a fad diet or fly by night plan, it is a lifestyle you can follow for the rest of your life to stay on the healthy highway.

C (carbs) - *make half your grains whole;* brown rice, oatmeal, corn tortilla, whole wheat tortillas, beans (black, kidney, pinto, white, etc.), potato, yam, grits, whole wheat bread, cream of wheat or rice

V (veggies) - *eat the rainbow;* asparagus, broccoli, pumpkin, squash, salads, beets, spinach, greens, zucchini, green peas, green beans, celery, carrots

F (fruit) - *make most choices whole fruit, not juice*; orange, watermelon, cantaloupe, grapefruit, banana, apple, pear, apricots, berries, and even dried fruits, like raisins, dates, etc.

D (Dairy) – *choose low-fat or non-fat milk (or soymilk) products;* milk, cheese, yogurt, cottage cheese, buttermilk

P (protein) – *go lean with protein*; chicken, eggs, turkey, fish, shrimp, whey protein powder, beans, hummus, nuts, seeds, peas & legumes

GF (good fats) - *some foods contain good fats*; these include walnuts, sunflower oil/ seeds, raw almonds, avocado, macadamia nut oil, ground flax seeds or oil, olive oil, pecans, almonds, salmon, mackerel, herring

****

Breakfast – P – D – C- GF- F
Eat something when you wake up (within one hour after rising)

Snack
Think simple: cheese and crackers, a handful of almonds & dried apricots, or a fruit and yogurt smoothie

Lunch – P-C-GF-V

Snack
Simple snack like fresh fruit (melon chunks), or carrot sticks and hummus dip

Dinner- P - GF – V – F –D? - C (some may want to avoid C at night)
Avoid eating anything 2 to 3 hours before going to bed at night.

Sleep

Sleep could be a chapter in its own right because we're talking about our bodies, our vehicles and all of our bodies need sleep and plenty of it. More sleep actually aids in weight loss and keeping it off. Sleep is very important for a healthy body, as well. Your car wouldn't run so well if you kept it on the road and didn't give it some good down time, would it? Your body is the same; it needs about seven or eight hours of sleep in a row to be a well-maintained machine. Your brain needs this down time the most. The standard seven to eight hours fluctuates between frames: some do fine on six, while others prefer nine. Even if you're older and think you don't need as much sleep, not so, your body and brain still need the rest. Children require even more sleep, including teenagers, so let them go ahead and sleep in every once in awhile.

Alcohol is not your friend for a good night's sleep; try to avoid it too close to bedtime. While it may help you relax after a rough day at work and make you feel a little drowsy before bed, it will also disrupt the REM (rapid eye movement) part of your sleep in the second half of the night, when most of the really deep sleep occurs. Likewise, exercise before bed can make it harder to fall asleep, because it reeves your body temperature and speeds up your heart rate. You should try to get your strenuous exercise in at least two hours before hitting the sack.

For a really well-oiled machine, try to go to bed and wake up at the same time every day, including weekends. The folks who do this seem to function better than the rest of us; they also adjust better when their nights are shortened by other events, like travel, family, work, etc. If you can't go to bed at the same time every night, waking up at the same time every day seems to be the most effective way to reset your body's clock and keep it ticking.

If you've been eating regular meals and snacks throughout the day, you may notice that you wake up after about four or five hours of sleep. This may be your body trying to keep that rhythm and is asking for breakfast. If you find this happens to you, try adding complex carbohydrates (something on your frame's grains or beans list) to your dinner (if you don't already). You may also find that a cup of warm milk or hot cocoa before bed helps you sleep through the night. By cocoa, I'm referring to rich, real chocolate without corn syrup. You've heard of milk and cookies before bed? You may have also heard that it's the amino acid tryptophan than helps this process. It's true; however it's in the milk. A nice glass of warm milk before bed helps your body relax and get ready for a long night's sleep. If you find your sleep disturbed in the night, speak to your doctor and also try a few natural remedies like warm milk before bed. A nice warm bath before bed is also a calming way to end the day and personally my favorite.

Affirmations

In our society we have been trained to have negative thoughts and feelings about ourselves and others. We often feel guilty about the choices we make, and there are even potato chips named "guilt free." I once heard someone say "guilt is a useless emotion." It may not be entirely useless, as I can think of a number of logical reasons to feel guilty, but eating a potato chip (or even a whole bag) is not one of them!

When you veer off the highway to health, realize you made a decision and then decide to make a better choice next time and get right back on the healthy highway. It's not about eating only what's perfectly healthy and "right", it's about feeling good. Sure, sometimes a hot fudge sundae or burger, fries and cola feel really good. Don't knock yourself down for the choices you made, it will only trigger a landslide of wrong turns because you attract what you think, and if you think guilt, more guilt is bound to come.

Repeat this saying out load:

"My body is a machine. This is the only body I will ever have, I am lucky to have been given it. I am happy to take care of it and treat it well so that it will carry me well throughout my lifetime."

How did that make you feel?

We need to recreate the image we have of ourselves and using daily affirmations is a good way to start. Make up your own, it can be short and simple or more detailed. Make it positive and in the present tense. Some affirmations to try are:

"I enjoy my food and eat as healthfully as possible."
"I take pride in my body and exercise every day."
"I deserve happiness and I am a good person."
"I quench my thirst with plenty of water."

Think positively and put yourself in a calm, relaxed state while you whole-heartedly repeat your affirmation. Being positive is the key, so if you feel like saying "I always overeat" stop yourself and say "I fill my body with healthy amounts of nutritious fuel."

It helps to visualize yourself doing what your words say. Repeat your affirmation and see yourself doing it. In high school I was on the track team, and our coach would instruct us to visualize being the first one to run over the finish line. The highway to health is similar: see yourself as the healthy, fit, person you want to be. Visualize yourself filling your tank with plenty of fruits, veggies and whole grains.

Love Yourself, Love Your Body

If there is one thing that you take away from this book, I hope it is that your body is an amazing machine, a one of a kind work of art, and a reflection of something grand and spectacular. Treat it that way and it will provide for you again and again.

There is a poem by Maya Angelou that I adore:

Love life, engage in it,
give it all you've got.
Love it with a passion,
because life truly does give back,
many times over,
what you put into it.

Now, in place of life add "*your body.*" Your body could one day save your life if it is well fueled and healthy. Remember to feel and express gratitude for your beautiful body. Your body is all yours, it is a wonderland, and you're so blessed to have it. Please let it know how much you care about it!

Thanks for cruising with me on the highway to health!

Resources

Below is a list of resources that may be of interest to someone wanting to learn more about creating a healthy lifestyle.

> *Diet for a New America*, John Robbins, 1987, this book completely rocked my world when I read it in 1989. The heir to the Baskin Robbins ice cream chain called out the atrocities of agribusiness and helped start another food revolution.

> *Diet for a Small Planet, Frances Moore Lappe,* 1971, quintessential book on the theory of vegetarianism and how changing what you eat can change your life and the world.

> *The Omnivore's Dilemma*, Michael Pollan, 2006, a startling look at America's current agribusinesses and the social, ethical, and environmental impact of four different meals.

> *Silent Spring*, Rachel Carson, 1962, this book called out the health and environmental risks associated to the use of pesticides. It is hailed as the forerunner in the environmental movement.

> Take your own *Portion Distortion* quiz online: http://hp2010.nhlbihin.net/portion

> For more information about the art and science of Ayurveda, see books with Ayurveda in the Bibliography or visit an Ayurvedic practitioner in your area. In Seattle, try *Life in Balance Ayurvedic Rejuvenation Center, or Wealth of Health* in Bellevue.

> For more information about bringing fresh local meat, dairy and produce to your community schools, visit:
>   o   The Edible School Yard at: www.edibleschoolyard.org
>   o   The Farm to School program: www.farmtoschool.org

> The books in the bibliography with asterisk (*) are recommended further reading and were major influences for me, personally and professionally.

Cook well, Eat well, Be Well

NOTES

Acknowledgements

I would like to start with huge thanks to you for caring enough about your body to take the time to read this book.

Writing this book has not only been a fabulous growing experience for me, but it truly feels like part of my calling. I am so grateful for the teachers, friends, family and colleagues who have helped me along the way.

My family has been tremendously supportive of me in the journey through this book. My mother, Janet, is an excellent proof reader, sounding board and beautiful inspiration for how beneficial it is to stay physically fit! She took up horseback riding at 60-something and is always eager to grow and try new things. She is proof that living a healthy lifestyle makes a difference as we grow older.

My sister, Becky, was an inspiration because she really wants to make the right choices and asks a lot of questions. I wanted to write a book that she and anyone else could turn to in order to get some questions answered and be armored with the ability to make the right choices!

Even though I'm a grown woman, I still think my big brother, David, is a super hero, he has rescued me again and again, and for that I will be eternally grateful. Thank you also to Randy who, years ago was an active listener when I first got the idea to write a book. My sweet little son, Cliff, couldn't be dearer to me, and for him and all his classmates, I write this so that their generation may be a healthy one.

My Editor-In-Chief, Helen, came through at the last minute: thank you more than words can say!

To Kurt, my long time friend and supporter, his illustrations and that of Valters were outstanding, thank you both so much for your time and effort. My dear friend, Kathy, you are about the best friend a person could ask for, thank you. To, Bard, whose generosity is amazing, he took me under his wing and for that I am indebted. Finally, Roger, who helped me with the finishing touches, thank you and then some!

Bibliography

Ayurvedic Remedies for the Whole Family, Dr. Light Miller; Lotus Press, Twin Lakes, WI, 1999.

Advertising in the United States, Anthony E. Gallo; Food Advertising USDA/ ERS AIB-750, Chapter 9. PDF format.

A Fresh Look at Food Preservatives; Judith E. Foulke, U. S. Food and Drug Administration, FDA Consumer, October 1993. http://www.cfsan.fda.gov/~dms/fdpreser.html - last accessed July 26, 2008.

Aim for a Healthy Weight; Obesity Education Initiative, National Heart, Lung and Blood Institute, United States Department of Health and Human Services and National Institute of Health, website: http://www.nhlbi.nih.gov/health/public/heart/obesity/lose_wt/risk.htm last accessed July 26, 2008.

American Dietetic Association website: http://www.eatright.org/cps/rde/xchg/ada/hs.xsl/index.html, last accessed on October 20, 2009.

Are Preservatives in Food Making Kids Hyper? Laura Sayre; Mother Earth News, April/May 2008, page 26.

Cereal Sales Soggy Despite Price Cuts and Reduced Couponing; Gregory K. Price, Structural Change in the U.S. Food Industry http://www.ers.usda.gov/publications/foodreview/may2000/may2000d.pdf last accessed on July 26, 2008.

Children's Life Expectancy Being Cut Short by Obesity; Pam Belluck, New York Times, March 17, 2005.

Concise Colour Medical Dictionary; Oxford University Press, Oxford, UK, 1998.

Cracking the Metabolic Code, James B. LaValle, R.Ph., C.C.N., N.D., with Stacy Lundin Yale, R.N., B.S.N., Basic Health Publications, Inc., 2004.

Curves Fitness & Weight Management Plan, Gary Heavin, Nadia Rodman, Cassie Findley, Curves International, Waco Tx, 2008.

Dietary Reference Intakes, Institute of Medicine, The National Academies Press, Washington, D.C., 2007.

*Feeding the Whole Family, Cynthia Lair, Sasquatch Books, Seattle, WA, 2008.

Fiber: Start roughing it! The Nutrition Source, Harvard School of Public Health, http://www.hsph.harvard.edu/nutritionsource/what-should-you-eat/fiber-full-story/index.html#intro last accessed on July 27, 2008.

Food Additives; U. S. Food and Drug Administration, FDA/IFIC Brochure: January 1992

Grading School Lunches; Taste for Life magazine, January 2008, page 11.

Health Care Savings Could Start in the Cafeteria, Melanie Warner, *The New York Times*, November 28, 2009.

Healthy Youth: An Investment in Our Nation's Future. U.S. Department of Health and Human Services, Centers for Disease Control and Prevention, 2003.

Introduction to Nutrition and Metabolism, 4th Edition; David A. Bender, CRC Press, Taylor & Francis Group, LLC, 2008.

Mayo Clinic on Digestive Health; John E. King, M.D., Mason Crest Publishers, Philadelphia, PA, 2000.

Media Smart Youth, Eat, Think and Be Active! A Workshop Curriculum for You Ages 11 to 13, Facilitator's Guide; U.S. Department of Heath and Human Services, National Institutes of Health, National Institutes of Child Health and Human Development, October 2005.

Northwest Health magazine; Rhonda Aronwald, Group Health, Winter, 2008, pages 2-3.

Ode Magazine, Mill Valley, CA, April 2008.

Our Big Problem, Theodore Dalrymple; *The Wall Street Journal*, W1, May 1-2, 2010.

Organic Agriculture, A Glossary of Terms for Farmers and Gardeners; Annie Eicher, Organic Farming Program Coordinator, University of California Davis Cooperative Extension, February 2003

On Food and Cooking, The Science and Lore of the Kitchen; Harold Mcgee, Collier Books, Macmillan Publishing Company, New York, 1984.

Pesticide Usage in the United States: History, Benefits, Risks, and Trends: Keith S. Delaplane, Professor of Entomology, The University of Georgia College of Agricultural and Environmental Sciences, Cooperative Extension Service, Bulletin 1121, November, 2000.

Science, Hill, J.O., Wyatt, H., et al, Volume 299, February 7, 2003.

Staying Healthy with Nutrition, 21st Century Edition, Elson M. Hass, MD, with Buck Levin, PhD, RD, Celestial Arts, 2006.

SuperFoods HealthStyle, Steven G. Pratt, M.D., and Kathy Matthews, William Morrow (HarperCollins), New York, NY, 2006.

The Allergy Exclusion Diet, Jill Carter and Alison Edwards, Hay House, Inc., Carlsbad, CA, 2002.

The Ayurvedic Cookbook, A Personalized Guide to Good Nutrition and Health, Amadea Morningstar and Urmila Desai; Lotus Press, Wilmot, WI, 1990.

The Body Sense Natural Diet, Lorna R. Vanderhaeghe, John Wiley & Sons Canada Ltd, Mississauga, Ontario, 2004.

The Buddha and His Sayings; Buddha Vachana Trust, Bangalore, India, 1989.

The Complete Fiber Fact Book, Rita Elkins, M.H., Woodland Publishing, Pleasant Grove, UT, 1999.

The Eighth Habit; Steven Covey, Free Press, FranklinCovey, Co., New York, NY, 2004

The Good Mood Diet, Susan Kleiner, PhD, RD, with Bob Condor, Springboard Press, NY, 2007.

The New Healing Foods, Coleen Pierre, M.S., R.D., American Master Products, Inc./Jerry Baker, USA, 2005.

The Sacred Kitchen, Higher Consciousness Cooking for Health and Wellness; Robin Robertson and Jon Robertson, New World Library, Novato, CA, 1999.

The Yoga of Herbs, An Ayurvedic Guide to Herbal Medicine, Dr. David Frawley and Dr. Vasant Lad; Lotus Press, Twin Lakes, WI, 1986.
Walk Your Way to Fitness, The Positive Line, Item # ITP-86, 2004.

6223136R0

Made in the USA
Charleston, SC
29 September 2010